Functional Training

ANATOMY

Kevin Carr

Mary Kate Feit, PhD

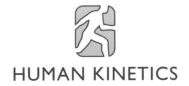

HUMAN KINETICS

Library of Congress Cataloging-in-Publication Data

Names: Carr, Kevin, 1987- author. | Feit, Mary Kate, 1988- author.
Title: Functional training anatomy / Kevin Carr, Mary Kate Feit.
Description: Champaign, IL : Human Kinetics, [2022]
Identifiers: LCCN 2020033351 (print) | LCCN 2020033352 (ebook) | ISBN
 9781492599104 (paperback) | ISBN 9781492599111 (epub) | ISBN
 9781492599135 (pdf)
Subjects: LCSH: Physical fitness. | Exercise. | Physical education and
 training.
Classification: LCC GV481 .C317 2022 (print) | LCC GV481 (ebook) | DDC
 613.7--dc23
LC record available at https://lccn.loc.gov/2020033351
LC ebook record available at https://lccn.loc.gov/2020033352

ISBN: 978-1-4925-9910-4 (print)

Acquisitions Editor: Michael Mejia; **Developmental Editor:** Amy Stahl; **Copyeditor:** Joyce Sexton; **Senior Graphic Designer:** Sean Roosevelt; **Cover Designer:** Keri Evans; **Cover Design Specialist:** Susan Rothermel Allen; **Photographs (cover and interior for illustration reference):** Bruce Carr; **Illustrator (cover):** Heidi Richter; **Photo Production Manager:** Jason Allen; **Senior Art Manager:** Kelly Hendren; **Illustrations:** © Human Kinetics/Heidi Richter and Jennifer Gibas; **Printer:** Versa Press

We thank Mike Boyle Strength and Conditioning in Woburn, Massachusetts, for assistance in providing the location for the photo shoot for this book.

Human Kinetics
1607 N. Market Street
Champaign, IL 61820
USA

United States and International
Website: **US.HumanKinetics.com**
Email: info@hkusa.com
Phone: 1-800-747-4457

Canada
Website: **Canada.HumanKinetics.com**
Email: info@hkcanada.com

E8107

Tell us what you think!
Human Kinetics would love to hear what we
can do to improve the customer experience.
Use this QR code to take our brief survey.

Functional Training

ANATOMY

CONTENTS

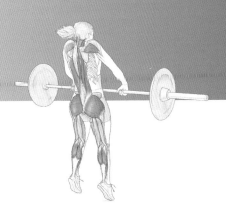

FOREWORD

Hiring Kevin Carr was probably the best decision I didn't make. It was the summer of 2010. Kevin Carr was a young intern from the University of Massachusetts. Nicole Rodriquez (our de facto head coach at the time) was gushing to me about Kevin and wanting to bring him back the next summer as an employee. My only words were "He's kind of quiet."

To be honest, I don't think I noticed Kevin much that first summer, but Nicole continued to rave about him. "He's going to be good," she said. I always trust my staff. They really do the hiring because they see how people work when I'm not around. (Just a reminder: That's really important.)

Fast-forwarding 10 years, I can safely say that bringing Kevin Carr back for another summer was one of the best non-decisions of my career. Kevin is now our business partner and the real driving force in the Certified Functional Strength Coach program. He's also a vital part of our business and is a big part of the future of Mike Boyle Strength and Conditioning.

I think the best way to describe Kevin is *a master learner.* He epitomizes the cliché about "getting a little better every day." Kevin just continues to improve as a coach, as a writer, as a speaker, and as a business person.

The highest compliment I can give to a person is that they *get it.* Kevin gets it. People might ask what *it* is. I'm not sure I can describe *it,* but I know it when I see it. What Kevin gets is people, timing, effort, integrity, and fun.

He's the perfect balance. Smart but not nerdy. Fit but not self-obsessed. Funny but not obnoxious. The truth is that Kevin Carr is the guy who makes a business owner say, "I wish I had 10 of those." If you've ever run a business, you know the kind of people I mean. They're the people who make your life easy. The people who do both the big and little things without being asked. The people you point out to other employees as examples of what you want.

Oh, yeah, and he wrote this book. Trust me: Kevin will deliver on this book the same way he delivers on everything else. Take the time to dig in. In 10 years, people will still be reading this book and talking about Kevin Carr, but at that point everyone will know his name. Keep reading—trust me.

Mike Boyle
Founder of Mike Boyle Strength and Conditioning

PREFACE

Ever since I (Kevin) began my coaching career at Mike Boyle Strength and Conditioning, I have made it my mission to improve the world's understanding of "functional training." At its most simple, functional training is purposeful training. It is training that is designed to support the human body in its daily demands, whether in activities of daily living or in the high-stress environment of competitive sports.

To understand functional training, you must first understand functional anatomy. Having a firm grasp of how the anatomy of the human body works is essential to building a complete functional training program. The way anatomy functions on a cadaver lying flat on a table is not an accurate representation of how the body functions while people are on their feet, moving dynamically. The context in which you learn anatomy matters, because it will directly reflect on practical application.

Many of the traditionalist approaches to strength training are based on "dead person anatomy," overly focused on single-joint, machine-centered exercises influenced by origin-insertion–based anatomy. Training influences from bodybuilding and powerlifting lead many athletes astray, such that they train solely for muscle size and strength with no thought of how this may translate to their sport. Functional training, instead, is based on living, moving anatomy with a focus on using multiplanar- and unilateral-based exercises with the goal of improving function and carryover to sport.

The goal in this book is to provide a functional, anatomical guide to efficient and effective training of the human body. Our hope is that athletes, coaches, and fitness enthusiasts will read this book and as a result have a better understanding of how to build a functional training program for themselves and others. The text in each chapter further explains the function of the anatomy shown in the illustrations. The anatomical illustrations that accompany the exercises are color coded to indicate the primary and secondary muscles and the connective tissues featured in each exercise.

☐ Primary muscles   ☐ Secondary muscles

Every exercise in chapters 2 through 8 includes three icons that represent the three planes of movement where an exercise may be performed—frontal, transverse, or sagittal. An icon or icons will be highlighted if that exercise is performed in the corresponding plane.

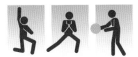

This book covers all aspects of a complete functional training program. We start by discussing the importance of mobility training and the impact that it has on movement quality, performance, and injury reduction. Next, we cover the use of movement preparation drills to improve movement efficiency and to warm up the body and prepare it for high-intensity activities. In chapter 4, we discuss how to perform and program plyometric and medicine ball exercises to train athletes to create and absorb force. In chapter 5, we cover heavy implement power development with the use of exercises like Olympic lifts and kettlebell swings. In the strength training portion of the book, we discuss all the movements that make up a complete training program, including hip-dominant, knee-dominant, pushing, pulling, and core exercises. In the final chapter, we show you how to put all these parts together to build a complete functional training program to reduce injuries and improve performance.

ACKNOWLEDGMENTS

Thank you to both of my parents for instilling in me a lifelong love of physical activity and exercise. I love you both.

Thank you to Mike Boyle, Bob Hanson, and all of the staff I have worked with at Mike Boyle Strength and Conditioning. I would not be where I am today if it had not been for your mentorship and friendship.

Kevin Carr

I want to thank Kevin for asking me to be part of this project. I'm happy that after more than a decade I am still part of the Mike Boyle Strength and Conditioning family.

I also want to thank my family. Adam, Cody, and Macy are my rocks. I wouldn't be able to do any of this without you!

Mary Kate Feit

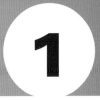

FUNCTIONAL TRAINING IN MOTION

In order to prepare properly to excel at your sport, you require a conscientiously designed training program that considers the optimal function of the human body. The idea of functional training is built on purposefully selecting the correct exercises based on your body's anatomical structure and function and on training the body with the goal of optimizing health and performance.

Whether you are an elite athlete or part of the general population, your program design and means of training should reflect the function of the human body and the demands that are placed upon it both in life and in the sporting arena. A functional training program should ensure that you have adequate joint mobility, movement quality, strength, power, and cardiovascular fitness to meet the demands of sport and life.

For the athletic population, functional training should safeguard athletes and improve performance in their sport. Many of the same mechanisms that will improve the athlete's performance will also reduce their likeliness of suffering injury. Improving active joint mobility will help the athlete to avoid strain and impingement injuries while also helping them to achieve the joint positions necessary to excel in the athletic tasks of their sport. The ability to run, jump, and throw reactively in a multitude of directions will improve the athlete's ability to be explosive on the field while also training them to absorb force efficiently to avoid deceleration related injuries. Developing full-body, multiplanar strength will also allow the athlete to absorb impact safely while also helping to produce power during athletic movements like running, jumping, swinging and throwing.

For the general population, functional training should improve people's ability to function in their everyday life and profession. Training should serve as a means to improve overall cardiovascular, metabolic, and neurological health. Training should improve people's ability to carry out daily tasks with vigor and alertness and should enhance their ability to safely participate in recreational activities.

Functional training, by definition, is a training intervention that helps the trainee function better, whether that means in everyday life or in competition. One should not view "functional training" as a special genre of training but as intelligent, purposeful training that is meant to restore movement quality, improve performance, and reduce the likeliness of injury.

FUNCTIONAL TRAINING IS COMPREHENSIVE TRAINING

A complete functional performance program should not just focus on the development of one single component but should strive to develop movement quality, strength, power, and cardiovascular fitness concurrently. The variable demands of most sporting environments and the interconnected nature of the human body require more than the expression of a singular capacity if one hopes to achieve success and longevity in sports and life.

An athlete who is strong but lacks mobility is at risk of muscle strains and joint damage. An athlete who is extremely mobile but is limited in strength will be overpowered by opponents and lack the ability to produce adequate levels of force. An athlete who is powerful but lacks aerobic conditioning will not be able to maintain power output over time and will fatigue prematurely.

A comprehensive, well-rounded functional training program should include all of the following components:

- Mobility training to optimize tissue extensibility and joint health
- Movement preparation drills to improve movement quality and efficiency
- Unilateral, bilateral, and multidirectional power exercises to develop deceleration skills and power expression
- Full-body strength exercises that address knee-dominant, hip-dominant, pushing, pulling, and core strengthening movement patterns and challenge the strength and stability of the body in multiple movement planes
- Energy system development that addresses the specific metabolic demands of the sport

This book provides a framework to assist you in selecting the most appropriate methods to train these components based on the anatomical structure and function of the human body. It will help you best understand exercise selection as well as some of the fundamental concepts that should guide your selection of specific exercises to improve human performance and reduce injuries.

PLANES OF MOTION IN THE HUMAN BODY

A well-designed functional training program should develop joint mobility, motor control, strength, and power in all three planes of movement to meet the variable movement demands of the sporting environment.

Three planes of motion are used to classify human movement: sagittal, frontal, and transverse (see figure 1.1). The *sagittal plane* divides the body laterally into right and left halves. Movements done in the sagittal plane are those in which the joints in the body move primarily anteriorly and posteriorly, with little to no intentional movement in the other planes of motion. The *frontal plane* divides the body anteriorly and posteriorly into front and back halves. Movements done in the frontal plane are those in which the majority of joint movement comes from moving from side to side. The *transverse plane* divides the body into top and bottom halves. Movements in the transverse plane are done rotationally.

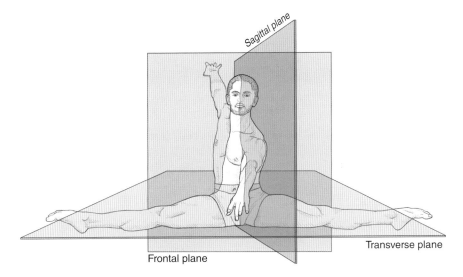

FIGURE 1.1 Three planes of movement.

This book covers exercises that address development of mobility, motor control, strength, and power in all of the planes to ensure balanced development of the athlete.

When discussing planar movement during exercise it is important to differentiate between *global planar movement* and *local planar forces* in relation to developing the local stabilizing musculature. Global planar movement describes where the majority of visual motion occurs during an exercise. Typically, global planar movement is controlled by the agonist or prime movers of the exercise. Local planar forces describe where isolated stabilizing actions must occur to complete the exercise successfully. Local planar forces are typically controlled by the synergists or stabilizing musculature.

During bilateral exercises like squats and deadlifts, the majority of motion occurs in the sagittal plane with minimal stability challenges occurring in the frontal and transverse planes. The balanced nature of a bilateral squat does not require frontal and transverse stabilizers of the hip and pelvis to work to maintain optimal alignment.

However, during unilateral exercises, in which work is being done by only one arm or one leg, the body must also stabilize in the frontal and transverse planes even when the majority of gross joint movement is occurring in the sagittal plane.

Take the example of a single-leg deadlift pattern (see figure 1.2). Even though the hip and knee joint are moving predominantly in the sagittal plane, the asymmetrical nature of unilateral exercise forces the dynamic stabilizers of the spine, pelvis, femur, tibia, and foot to control proper joint position, balance, and posture.

When selecting exercises in a functional training program, you want to take into consideration the local planar forces that are being exerted to ensure you develop the stabilizing musculature that is required for dynamic postural control. The development of multiplanar stability is vital for performance and injury reduction in a sporting environment.

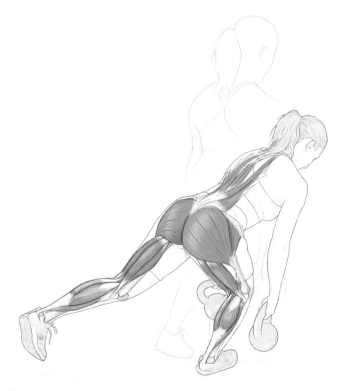

FIGURE 1.2   During the single-leg deadlift the gluteus medius, adductors, and obliques must work to stabilize the pelvis and femur in the frontal and transverse planes while the hamstrings, gluteus maximus, and spinal erectors work as prime movers in the sagittal plane.

FUNCTIONAL TRAINING REQUIRES FUNCTIONAL ANATOMY

The body has evolved to develop a great many interconnected systems that allow people to move dynamically throughout daily life. An athlete's ability to run, jump, and throw can be attributed to the body's amazing network of bones, muscles, tendons, and fasciae that allow them to flex, extend, and rotate as an integrated unit and produce force with a single coordinated outcome.

Although people are traditionally taught strength training and anatomy in isolation, single-muscle functions and single-joint exercise do not accurately represent real-life movement. Nothing in the body occurs in a silo. The body functions as an interconnected unit, all pieces interdependent on one another, constantly adjusting function to carry out the desired task. In designing functional training programs, one must take into consideration not just the anatomy of the human body but also how anatomy functions in an integrated way in specific sporting environments.

Consider the function of the hamstring muscles during running. Traditionally one is taught that the biceps femoris, semimembranosus, and semitendinosus muscles function primarily as knee flexors—and in an isolated setting, such as on a leg curl machine, they would.

However, when you consider the function of a hamstring when you are on your feet, standing, running, or walking, the functionality of the hamstring is much different. A biarticular muscle group, crossing both the hip and knee, the hamstring muscles must carry out numerous actions during the gait cycle in conjunction with the obliques and glutes (see figure 1.3).

Functionally, the hamstrings serve in the following ways:

- As concentric hip extensors assisting the glutes during the takeoff phase of running
- As isometric stabilizers of pelvis assisting the obliques to maintain posterior pelvic tilt
- As eccentric decelerators of knee extension at the end of the forward swing phase

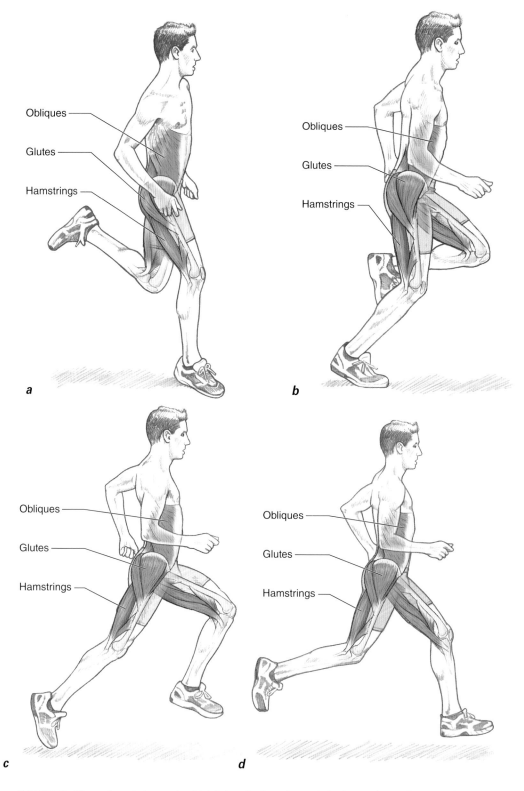

FIGURE 1.3   The gait cycle in running highlights the functions of the hamstrings, glutes, and obliques: (a) initial contact, (b) stance phase, (c) takeoff, and (d) forward swing phase.

Understanding functional anatomy as it relates to sport can help you select exercises that improve performance and reduce injury. In this specific instance, you would want to select hamstring exercises that train the hamstring as a hip extensor, pelvic stabilizer, and eccentric knee extender rather than primarily as a concentric knee flexor. A great exercise choice would be the single-leg deadlift or the sliding leg curl from chapter 7 rather than a traditional machine-based hamstring curl.

TRADITIONAL TRAINING VERSUS FUNCTIONAL TRAINING

Traditional performance programs that have been strongly influenced by bodybuilding and powerlifting often place a large emphasis on bilateral and machine-based strength exercises. And although many bilateral exercises like goblet squats and trap bar deadlifts (both in chapter 7) are valuable and should be used in a functional training program, you should look to prioritize developing strength unilaterally, in an attempt to represent the way the body moves in everyday life as well as in sporting activities.

Machine-based training often focuses on isolated movements that do not require the body to create stability authentically and that fail to accurately represent the stressors of real-life movement. While this approach may be valuable for targeted hypertrophy (muscle growth), it should be avoided in the development of a functional training program.

Traditional bilateral-based lifts like the squat, bench press, and deadlift can be valuable tools to develop fundamental sagittal plane strength and stability. However, after achieving entry-level competency, you should progress, using a complete functional program, from classic powerlifting- and bodybuilding-influenced lifts to unilateral exercises that challenge stability in the frontal and transverse planes.

ANTERIOR AND POSTERIOR OBLIQUE SYSTEMS

The human body has evolved to function unilaterally. Neurologically, humans are wired to walk, run, leap, and crawl in contralateral patterns. Consequently, the structural design of muscles, tendons, and fasciae has evolved to support the body's unilateral function.

The body has developed an intricate force-producing and stabilizing system known as the *anterior and posterior oblique system* (see figure 1.4), created by a continuum of muscles and fasciae, that runs across the body, allowing people to run, jump, and throw with amazing amounts of capacity and variability.

The discovery of the anterior and posterior oblique systems revealed how force is transferred across the body in both the transverse and frontal planes to produce power and stability in sport.

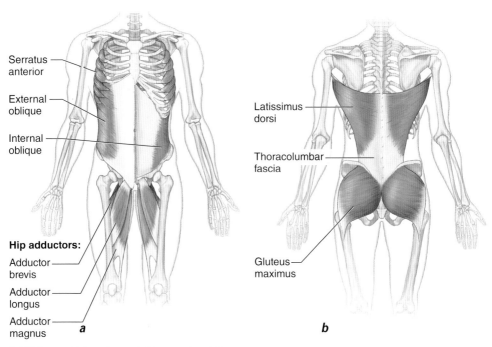

Serratus anterior

External oblique

Internal oblique

Hip adductors:

Adductor brevis

Adductor longus

Adductor magnus

a

Latissimus dorsi

Thoracolumbar fascia

Gluteus maximus

b

FIGURE 1.4   *(a)* Anterior and *(b)* posterior oblique systems.

Following the spiral lines of the body (see figure 1.5), you can see clearly how force produced on one side of the body can be transferred up the interconnected chain of muscles, tendons, and bones to the opposite side of the body.

The muscles and fasciae that make up the spiraling system of the anterior and posterior oblique systems are what allow you to create powerful, efficient, and coordinated actions like throwing a ball, swinging a golf club, leaping into the air, swinging a tennis racket, or bracing against contact from another competitor. Even mundane daily actions like reaching into a cabinet, stepping over an object, or getting up from a chair rely on the interconnected makeup of our muscular system.

To most effectively train the human body, it is recommended that you prioritize unilateral approaches to target the body's contralateral design. Looking at figure 1.6, you can see how during the single-leg squat the body relies heavily on coactivation of the muscles in the anterior and posterior oblique systems.

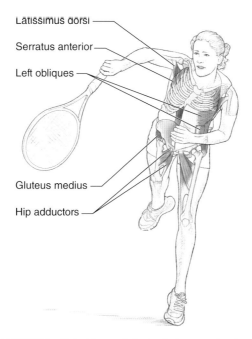

Latissimus dorsi

Serratus anterior

Left obliques

Gluteus medius

Hip adductors

FIGURE 1.5   Spiral lines of the body in a tennis player.

When you pick one foot up off the ground to perform a single-leg squat, the planar nature of squatting completely changes. The exercise starts with a bilateral squat, a predominantly sagittal plane exercise, and moves to a single-leg squat in which you immediately must demonstrate frontal and transverse plane control using the oblique systems to stabilize and propel through the movement.

When performing a single-leg squat on the left leg, you propel upward using the left glute, adductors, and hamstrings while stabilizing over the single support leg using the thoracolumbar fascia, contralateral quadratus lumborum, and external obliques. These are the same systems that are in use every time you strike the ground with a single foot on the field of play, safeguarding you from an injury.

You can identify these same spiral patterns when recognizing how athletes produce power and stabilize when swinging a racket, throwing a ball, or executing simple tasks of daily living.

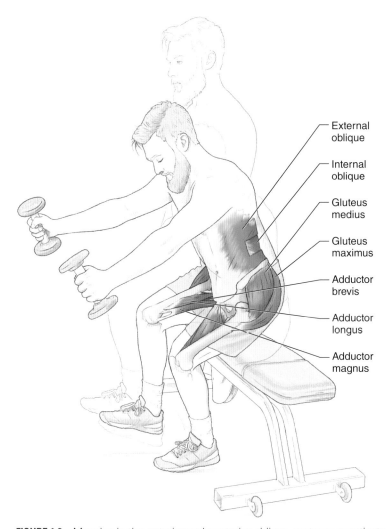

External
oblique

Internal
oblique

Gluteus
medius

Gluteus
maximus

Adductor
brevis

Adductor
longus

Adductor
magnus

FIGURE 1.6 Muscles in the anterior and posterior oblique systems coactivate during the single-leg squat.

The amazing tensegrity model that is the human body can coordinate powerful, accurate, and controlled sporting movements because it operates as a tightly interconnected system. The body's network of bones, muscles, tendons, and fasciae is controlled and integrated by the nervous system.

The human body functions as a multidirectional network, in which the whole functions better than the sum of its individual parts. It is essential to consider how the human anatomy functions synchronously as a system, in a dynamic sporting environment, when you select exercises to build a functional performance program. The following chapters of this text offer a framework that will guide you to create a functional training program based on the body's functional anatomy.

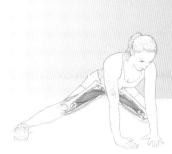

2

MOBILITY
EXERCISES

The first priority in any functional training program is that all your joints can move through a full range of motion with no pain or limitations. Limitations in joint mobility due to tissue stiffness can often lead to compensatory movement strategies and degeneration of the joint surface.

MOBILITY AND FLEXIBILITY

Joint mobility is the ability of a joint to actively move through a given range of motion. In training, your goal should be to maximize your active range of motion in all the major joints.

On reading this definition, you might think *mobility* means the same thing as *flexibility,* but functionally these two words have different definitions:

- *Flexibility* refers to the passive range of motion of a given joint and surrounding soft tissue structures.
- *Mobility* refers to the active range of motion and neurological control of a given joint and surrounding soft tissue structures.

While the differences between flexibility and mobility may not seem substantial, the difference between their effects on functionality could not be more profound. To have a truly functional, efficiently moving body, you should strive for both flexibility and mobility.

During loaded movement, muscles do not simply stretch passively; they must lengthen under eccentric tension, using tensile strength and neurological control of the joint. When a muscle is stretched under load, its ability to do so without rupture is not just a function of its flexibility, but also of local muscular strength and control of the movement via the nervous system. Consider a baseball player reaching up to make a catch to rob the opposing team of a home run. While it is important for the player to have the passive mobility to reach his arm overhead, he must also have the neurological control and tissue strength in the muscles of the shoulder complex to decelerate the movement to avoid shoulder dislocation or soft tissue injury. It is not enough to place passive stretches onto tissues to create useful range of motion; it is also necessary to actively produce muscular force while stretching to change tissue structure and create neurological control.

The exercise instruction portion of this chapter provides cueing on how to actively pursue joint mobility for maximal movement quality and injury reduction.

MOBILITY AND REGIONAL INTERDEPENDENCE

Health and functionality of the body relies heavily on the ability of joints to get into proper position to absorb and adapt to stress. As training stress increases due to limited recovery or to greater training volume, the resting neurological tension of the connective tissues often increases, limiting the degrees of freedom in the joint. If left unchecked, limitations in joint mobility can lead to joint degradation, connective tissue injuries, and compensatory movement strategies.

It is paramount to maintain the function of each joint in the body on an isolated level before effectively initiating traditional full-body exercises. Without adequate range of motion and neurological control at one joint, you are likely to compensate at adjacent joints to make up for that lack of range of motion. The body is regionally interdependent, with each joint system relying on the proper function of the joint systems above and below it. Limitations in function at one joint often lead the body to seek less efficient movement strategies in an effort to successfully complete a movement task.

For example, if you lack ankle dorsiflexion during a squat, you will have to make up for that limitation in mobility by substituting adduction of the big toe, excessive pronation of the foot, internal rotation of the tibia, and adduction of the femur, often placing excessive valgus stress on the medial structure of the knee (see figure 2.1).

Maintaining adequate mobility in all of the body's joints ensures that sufficient degrees of freedom are present to move through full ranges of motion without placing undue stress on the joint and surrounding connective tissue or driving compensatory movement strategies in the neighboring joint systems.

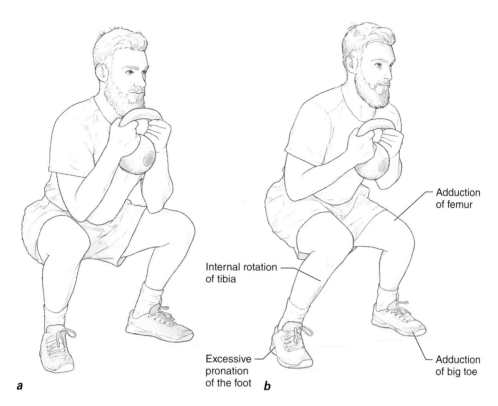

Adduction
of femur

Internal rotation
of tibia

Excessive
pronation
of the foot

Adduction
of big toe

a   *b*

FIGURE 2.1   *(a)* Squat using proper technique and adequate mobility versus *(b)* compensated squat.

90/90 HIP STRETCH (EXTERNAL ROTATION AND FLEXION FOCUS)

MOBILITY

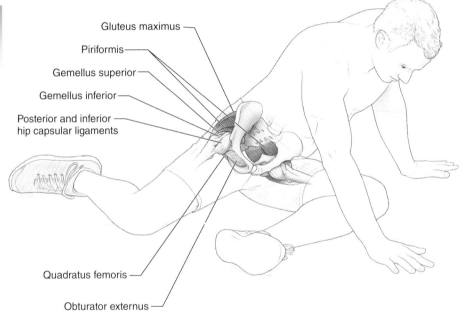

Gluteus maximus

Piriformis

Gemellus superior

Gemellus inferior

Posterior and inferior hip capsular ligaments

Quadratus femoris

Obturator externus

Execution

1. Sit on the ground with your hips, knees, and ankles all at right angles. Position one leg in front and one leg behind you.
2. Position your hands on either side of your front, externally rotated leg.
3. Actively press your front leg down into the ground by contracting the glute on the front leg.
4. Actively use your hip flexor to pull your torso over your front leg while maintaining a neutral spine. Repeat on the opposite side.

Muscles Involved

Primary:

- Posterior and inferior hip capsular ligaments
- Gluteus maximus
- Piriformis

Secondary:

- Gemellus superior and inferior
- Obturator externus
- Quadratus femoris

(continued)

90/90 HIP STRETCH (EXTERNAL ROTATION AND FLEXION FOCUS) *(continued)*

VARIATION

90/90 Hip Stretch (Internal Rotation and Extension Focus)

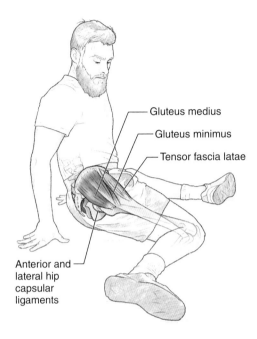

Gluteus medius

Gluteus minimus

Tensor fascia latae

Anterior and lateral hip capsular ligaments

This variation of the 90/90 hip stretch is done to focus on developing internal rotation and extension of the hip joint. This exercise is done in the same seated 90/90 position as the main exercise; however, the focus is on stretching the opposite hip into internal rotation and extension.

Sit on the ground with your hips, knees, and ankles all at right angles. Position one leg in front of you and one leg behind you. Position your hands on either side of your hips, sitting up as tall as possible. Actively press both legs down into the ground. Actively pull your torso toward your rear, internally rotated leg.

SPIDERMAN STRETCH

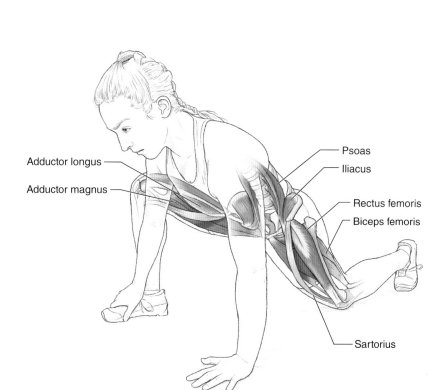

Adductor longus

Adductor magnus

Psoas

Iliacus

Rectus femoris

Biceps femoris

Sartorius

(continued)

MOBILITY

SPIDERMAN STRETCH   *(continued)*

Execution

1. Start in the top of a push-up position with your hands directly under your shoulders.
2. Step your right foot forward so that it is outside of your right hand and drop your left knee down to the ground.
3. Drive your right elbow into your right knee while pressing back into your elbow using your adductor musculature.
4. Drive your rear hip down toward the floor using your glute muscles. Repeat on the opposite side.

Muscles Involved

Primary:

- Adductor magnus
- Adductor longus
- Semimembranosus
- Semitendinosus
- Gracilis (front hip)
- Anterior capsular ligaments
- Iliacus
- Psoas
- Rectus femoris (rear hip)

Secondary:

- Biceps femoris (front hip)
- Sartorius (rear hip)

FUNCTIONAL FOCUS

The spiderman stretch is a dual-purpose mobility drill to improve mobility of the lead hip into flexion and the rear hip into extension. This drill is particularly effective at improving hip mobility for squatting on the lead hip while improving hip extension in the rear hip for activities such as sprinting. Lack of hip mobility can negatively affect sprinting form and lead to compensatory movements through the spine and pelvis, leading to back pain.

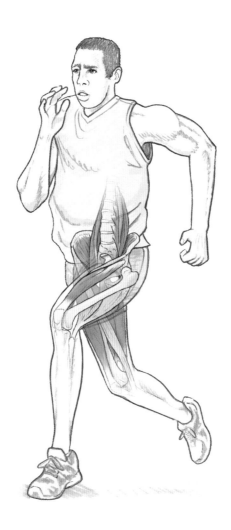

STRAIGHT-LEG ADDUCTOR ROCKING

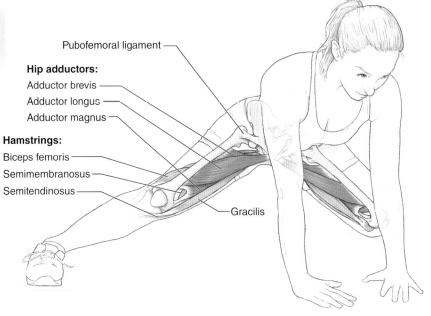

Pubofemoral ligament

Hip adductors:
Adductor brevis
Adductor longus
Adductor magnus

Hamstrings:
Biceps femoris
Semimembranosus
Semitendinosus

Gracilis

Execution

1. Start in a kneeling position with your hips abducted apart as far as possible.
2. Straighten your right leg to the side so that your knee is extended, ankle is inverted, and your foot is flat on the ground.
3. While maintaining a flat spine, drive your hips backward toward the ground behind you while actively exhaling out of the mouth.
4. Rock forward and repeat for the programmed repetitions. Repeat on the opposite side.

Muscles Involved

Primary:

- Pubofemoral ligament
- Hip adductors (adductor longus, adductor magnus, adductor brevis)

Secondary:

- Gracilis
- Pectineus
- Hamstrings (semitendinosus, semimembranosus, biceps femoris)

(continued)

MOBILITY

STRAIGHT-LEG ADDUCTOR ROCKING   *(continued)*

FUNCTIONAL FOCUS

Straight-leg adductor rocking is effective at improving tissue extensibility into hip abduction. Having adequate frontal plane hip mobility is especially important for change of direction in field- and court-based sports as well as in skating sports. Lack of hip adduction tissue extensibility can put athletes at risk for adductor strains and sports hernia injuries.

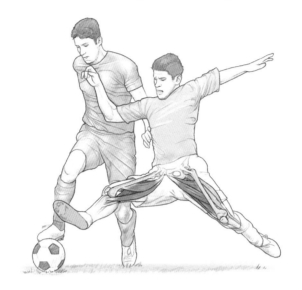

HALF-KNEELING HIP FLEXOR STRETCH

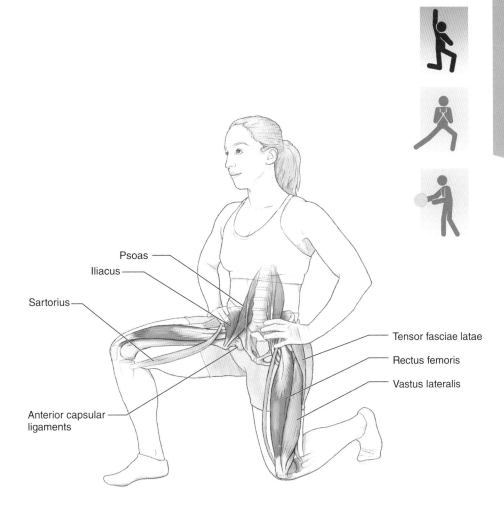

Psoas

Iliacus

Sartorius

Tensor fasciae latae

Rectus femoris

Vastus lateralis

Anterior capsular ligaments

(continued)

HALF-KNEELING HIP FLEXOR STRETCH *(continued)*

Execution

1. Start in a half-kneeling position with your left knee down and your right leg out in front with your knee at a 90-degree angle.
2. Dorsiflex your left ankle so that your toes dig into the ground.
3. Focus on posteriorly tilting your pelvis and drawing your ribs downward to create tension in your abdomen.
4. Maintain abdominal tension while contracting your glute and actively diaphragmatically breathing into the nose and out of the mouth. Repeat on opposite site.

Muscles Involved

Primary:

- Anterior capsular ligaments
- Iliacus
- Psoas
- Rectus femoris

Secondary:

- Vastus lateralis
- Tensor fasciae latae
- Sartorius

FUNCTIONAL FOCUS

The purpose of the half-kneeling hip flexor stretch is to improve tissue extensibility through the anterior hip musculature, specifically the iliacus, psoas, and rectus femoris. It is especially important to maintain hip extension mobility to protect hip health when participating in sports that require a high volume of hip flexion, like sprinting, cycling, and skating sports.

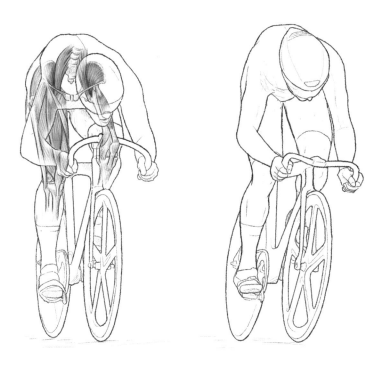

WALL QUAD STRETCH

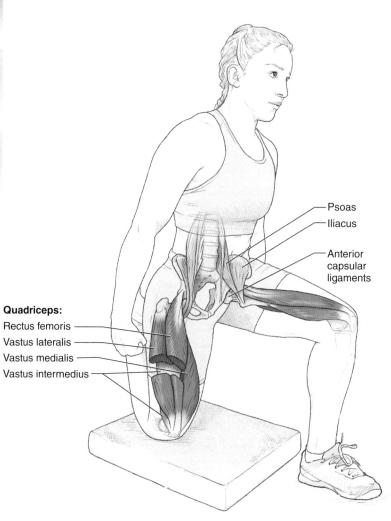

Psoas

Iliacus

Anterior
capsular
ligaments

Quadriceps:
Rectus femoris
Vastus lateralis
Vastus medialis
Vastus intermedius

Execution

1. In a half-kneeling position, wedge your right knee up against a wall with your back to the wall. Bend your right leg at the knee, so your foot is between the wall and your bottom. You may place your knee on a mat for comfort.

2. Your left leg should be in front of your body with your knee at a 90-degree angle and your foot flat on the floor.

3. Extend your hips and spine so that you are sitting up tall with a straight line between your knee and your head.

4. Maintain a posterior pelvic tilt and abdominal tension while actively diaphragmatically breathing into the nose and out of the mouth.

Muscles Involved

Primary:

- Anterior capsular ligaments
- Quadriceps (rectus femoris, vastus lateralis, vastus medialis, vastus intermedius)

Secondary:

- Iliacus
- Psoas

(continued)

WALL QUAD STRETCH   *(continued)*

FUNCTIONAL FOCUS

Lack of quadriceps flexibility can limit heel height recovery during sprinting and increase the likelihood of patellar femoral pain. Improvements in quadriceps flexibility from mobility training can allow for better sprinting mechanics and reduce instances of quadriceps strains and knee pain.

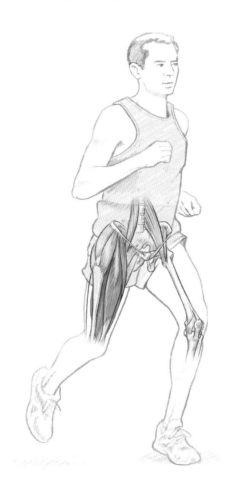

ANKLE DORSIFLEXION

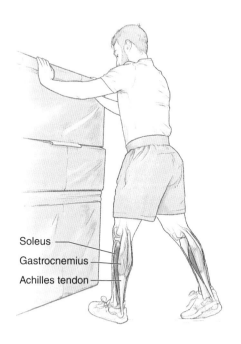

Soleus
Gastrocnemius
Achilles tendon

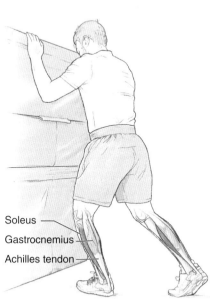

Soleus
Gastrocnemius
Achilles tendon

(continued)

ANKLE DORSIFLEXION   *(continued)*

Execution

1. Stand 1 foot (0.3 m) away from a wall or wall of mats with your palms firmly planted on the wall.
2. Stagger your feet and load 90 percent of your weight onto your lead leg.
3. Drive the back knee directly over the middle of the foot, past the toes as far as you can without picking up your front heel. Actively pull yourself into dorsiflexion by contracting your anterior tibialis.
4. Hold this position for 10 seconds and repeat for the programmed repetitions. Repeat on the opposite side.

Muscles Involved

Primary:

- Achilles tendon
- Soleus

Secondary:

- Gastrocnemius

FUNCTIONAL FOCUS

Ankle dorsiflexion is extremely important for sprinting and deceleration in sport as well as for proper squatting and lunging form in the weight room. A lack of ankle dorsiflexion leaves athletes at risk for ankle sprains and soft tissue ruptures to the soleus, gastrocnemius, Achilles tendon, and plantar fascia.

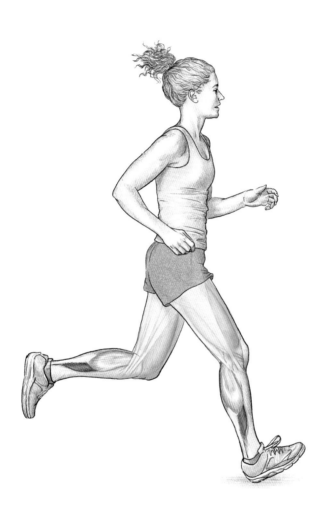

SHOULDER-CONTROLLED ARTICULAR ROTATION (FLEXION FOCUS)

MOBILITY

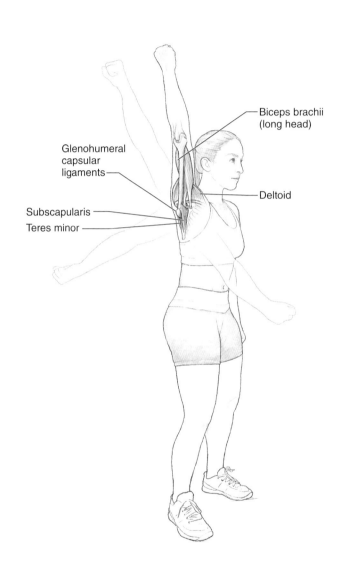

Biceps brachii (long head)

Glenohumeral capsular ligaments

Deltoid

Subscapularis

Teres minor

Execution

1. Stand next to a wall, roughly 1 foot (0.3 m) away, with the lateral aspect of your shoulder facing the wall.

2. With your elbow straight and your arm fully supinated and externally rotated, flex the shoulder up as high as you can without compensating with extension and rotation in the thorax.

3. Upon reaching end range, internally rotate and pronate the arm and continue circumduction behind your body until you return to the start position.

4. This drill should be done slowly and under control, with full muscular tension around the joint and no compensatory movement through the thorax. Perform for five repetitions before repeating on the opposite side.

Muscles Involved

Primary:
- Glenohumeral capsular ligaments

Secondary:
- Deltoid
- Biceps brachii (long head)
- Rotator cuff (infraspinatus, supraspinatus, subscapularis, teres minor)

(continued)

SHOULDER-CONTROLLED ARTICULAR ROTATION (FLEXION FOCUS)   *(continued)*

VARIATION

Shoulder-Controlled Articular Rotation (Extension Focus)

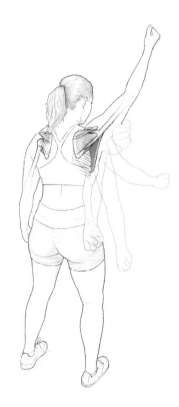

This variation of shoulder-controlled articular rotation of the glenohumeral joint focuses on developing global circumduction into extension. Stand next to a wall, roughly 1 foot (0.3 m) away, with the lateral aspect of your shoulder facing the wall. With your elbow straight and your arm fully pronated and internally rotated, extend the shoulder back as far as you can without compensating with flexion and rotation in the thorax. Upon reaching end range, externally rotate and supinate the arm and continue circumduction until you return to the start position. This drill should be done slowly and under control with full muscular tension around the joint and no compensation through the thorax. Perform for five repetitions before repeating on the opposite side.

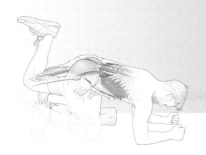

MOTOR CONTROL AND MOVEMENT PREPARATION EXERCISES

3

Movement preparation drills are exercises used during the warm-up to teach athletes how to move most efficiently and prepare the body for higher-intensity exercises in the training program. These exercises improve and develop motor control, which is the ability of an individual to control movement through neurological pathways. Assuming you possess the joint mobility necessary to complete a movement pattern, you want to work on developing your ability to efficiently move through that range of motion under low load before progressively loading within the strength program. Simply put, you need to learn how to move the right joints, using the right muscles at the right time.

Often athletes exhibit inefficient compensatory movement strategies that can leave them at higher risk for injury in training and competition. An example might be the substitution of lumbar extension as compensation for lack of hip extension or lack of core stability (or both). Compensatory strategies like this can lead to overuse of the compensating muscle group, local joint degeneration, and fatigue. By progressively retraining movement patterns, you will become efficient and will lessen the likelihood of injury and biomechanical breakdown over time.

Ideally, you want to select movement drills in this section that will directly correlate to the exercises you intend to use in the strength and power portion of the training program, as well as correlate to your sport's specific performance. By using low-threshold movement preparation drills that carry over to high-threshold strength and power drills, you can ensure movement efficiency before adding load and speed to the movement pattern.

Following is an example of the progressive connection between movement preparation drills and strength and power exercises in a functional training program.

The leg lower is used to develop pelvic stability and improve opposing hip flexion and extension (see figure 3.1). The leg lower trains the abdominal musculature to stabilize the pelvis, reducing the resting tone in the hip flexors and hamstrings and allowing for greater expression of hip flexion and extension range of motion. The ability to access full hip flexion and extension is vital in running as well as in the ability to execute exercises like the single-leg deadlift (see chapter 1).

The single-leg deadlift is a strength exercise that develops posterior chain strength and multiplanar hip stability. Performing it properly requires the ability to demonstrate full hip flexion and extension and thus is supported by movement preparation drills like the leg lower, shown in figure 3.1.

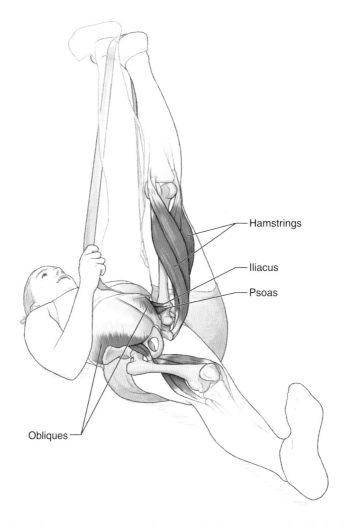

FIGURE 3.1   The leg lower is used to develop pelvic stability to improve opposing hip flexion and extension during hinging exercises like the single-leg deadlift.

Actions like planting a foot at high speed to kick a soccer ball require an extreme amount of hip mobility and stability (see figure 3.2). To functionally support this activity on the field, you should use the leg lower to improve hip range of motion and the single-leg deadlift to develop hip stability.

It is important to achieve joint positions under low-load and low-stress conditions before performing high-load and high-velocity activities. As stated earlier, motor control drills can develop efficient movement strategies and help you to warm up before moving on to higher-intensity training.

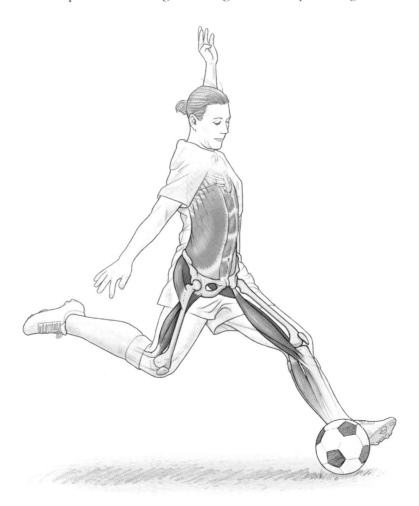

FIGURE 3.2 The athlete must be strong enough to stabilize her plant leg while maximally separating her hips without compensating at her lumbar spine.

SUPINE DIAPHRAGMATIC BREATHING

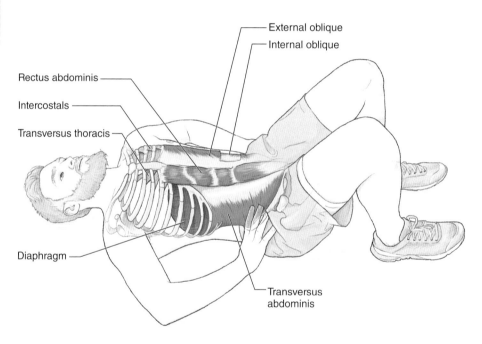

Execution

1. Lie flat on your back with your knees bent and feet flat on the floor.
2. Slightly posteriorly tilt your pelvis so that your spine is flat on the floor and your tailbone is elevated.
3. Inhale through the nose for four seconds, expanding your thorax in all directions.
4. Exhale through the mouth for eight seconds, drawing your rib cage down and inward. Hold your breath at the end for two seconds.

Muscles Involved

Primary:

- Diaphragm
- Rectus abdominis
- Internal oblique
- External oblique
- Transversus abdominis

Secondary:

- Transversus thoracis
- Intercostals

(continued)

SUPINE DIAPHRAGMATIC BREATHING *(continued)*

FUNCTIONAL FOCUS

The purpose of diaphragmatic breathing drills is to train athletes' ability to recruit their fundamental respiratory musculature. Proper use of the diaphragm and internal and external obliques will promote improved gas exchange during ventilation as well as improve core stability and positioning of the rib cage and pelvis during exercise.

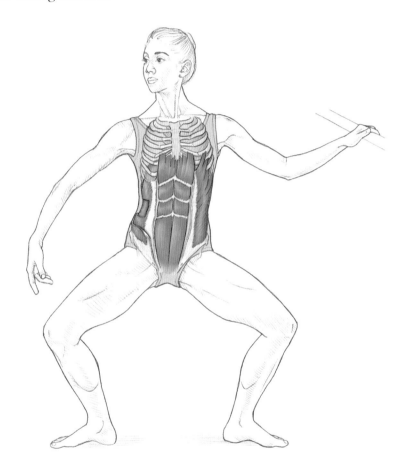

FLOOR SLIDE

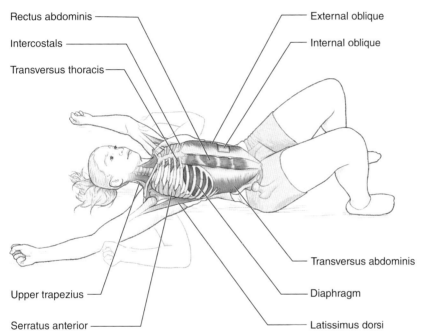

Rectus abdominis

Intercostals

Transversus thoracis

External oblique

Internal oblique

Upper trapezius

Serratus anterior

Transversus abdominis

Diaphragm

Latissimus dorsi

(continued)

FLOOR SLIDE *(continued)*

Execution

1. Lie flat on your back with your knees bent and feet flat on the floor, with your shoulders externally rotated and arms in a W position on the floor beside you.

2. Slightly posteriorly tilt your pelvis so that your spine is flat on the floor and your tailbone is elevated.

3. Before beginning the exercise, inhale through the nose. Exhale through the mouth while sliding the arms overhead as far as possible and maintaining ground contact with fists and elbows.

4. Inhale while returning the elbows to the start position. Maintain contact of lumbar spine with the ground throughout the entire drill.

Muscles Involved

Primary:

- Diaphragm
- Rectus abdominis
- Internal oblique
- External oblique
- Transversus abdominis
- Teres minor
- Infraspinatus
- Supraspinatus

Secondary:

- Transversus thoracis
- Intercostals
- Latissimus dorsi
- Serratus anterior
- Upper and lower trapezius

FUNCTIONAL FOCUS

The floor slide is used to develop proper motor control sequencing of the humerus, scapula, and rib cage while performing overhead flexion and external rotation of the shoulder. When athletes have limited shoulder mobility and poor anti-extension control of the torso, they often substitute trunk extension for shoulder flexion, leaving them at risk for shoulder impingement or neck and shoulder pain due to compensatory movement strategies. This drill teaches you to achieve flexion and external rotation of the humerus and upward rotation of the scapula while maintaining rib cage depression and internal rotation. Improvements in this drill will support proper form in overhead drills like throwing, overhead presses, and pull-ups.

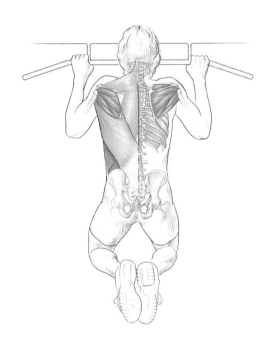

(continued)

FLOOR SLIDE   *(continued)*

VARIATION

Wall Slide

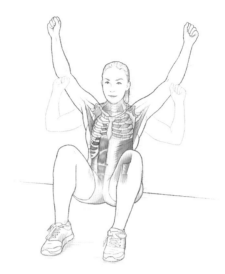

Sit against the base of a wall with your knees bent, feet flat, and your head and spine pressed flat against the wall. Externally rotate your shoulders into a W-shaped position so that the back of your hands, forearms, and shoulders are pressed against the wall. Before beginning the drill, inhale through the nose. Exhale through the mouth while sliding the arms overhead as far as possible while actively externally rotating the shoulders and maintaining contact against the wall with the lumbar spine, fists, and forearms. Inhale while returning the elbows to the start position. Maintain contact of lumbar spine, forearms, and hands with the wall throughout the entire drill.

The wall slide is a progression of the floor slide, made more challenging due to the vertical positioning of the torso. In progressing from supine to vertical, you must now stabilize the spine in the sagittal plane without the support of the ground. The drill is also more difficult because in moving to a vertical position you are no longer assisted by gravity to externally rotate the shoulder, and you now must actively externally rotate the shoulder to maintain contact with the wall.

LEG LOWER WITH BAND STABILIZATION

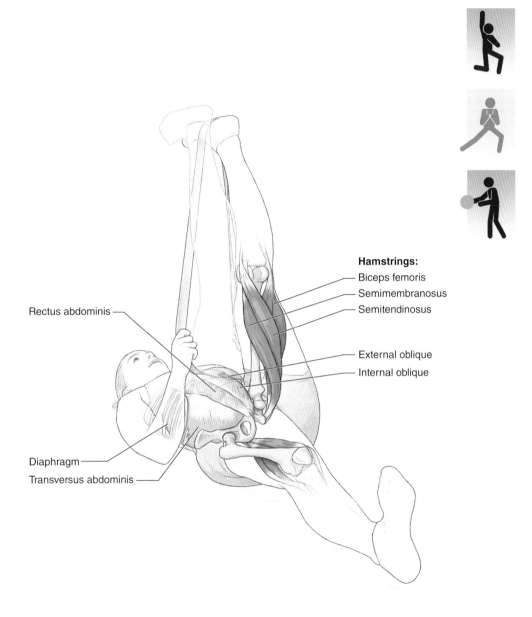

Hamstrings:
Biceps femoris
Semimembranosus
Semitendinosus

External oblique
Internal oblique

Rectus abdominis

Diaphragm
Transversus abdominis

(continued)

LEG LOWER WITH BAND STABILIZATION *(continued)*

Execution

1. Lie on your back with your knees straight and a band in your hands and around the arch of one foot.

2. Flex your hips, bringing your legs as high as possible while keeping your knees straight.

3. Inhale through your nose before beginning the exercise. Exhale through your mouth as you slowly lower the leg without the band toward the ground, keeping the knee straight.

4. Keep the leg with the band completely still and straight throughout the drill. Inhale as you return the other leg to the top position. Repeat on the opposite side.

Muscles Involved

Primary:

- Hamstrings (semitendinosus, semimembranosus, biceps femoris)

Secondary:

- Rectus abdominis
- Diaphragm
- Internal oblique
- External oblique
- Transversus abdominis

FUNCTIONAL FOCUS

The leg-lowering progression is used to develop opposing hip flexion and extension. The ability to simultaneously flex and extend the hips through a full range of motion allows you to run and hinge without compensatory motions through the spine and pelvis that could lead to injury and limit performance. Once you demonstrate competency with the band-assisted variations, you should progress to the unassisted variation to further develop trunk, pelvic, and femoral motor control.

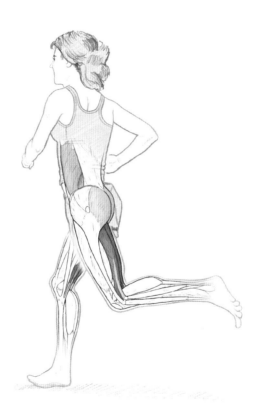

(continued)

LEG LOWER WITH BAND STABILIZATION   *(continued)*

VARIATION

Unassisted Leg Lower

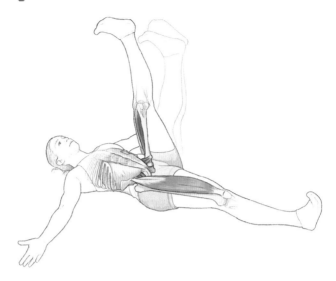

Lie on your back with both knees straight and hips flexed straight up in the air as high as possible. Inhale through your nose before beginning the exercise. Exhale through your mouth as you slowly lower one leg toward the ground, keeping the knee straight. Keep the stationary leg completely still and straight, actively flexing it up throughout the drill. Inhale as you return the moving leg to the top position. Repeat on the opposite side.

QUADRUPED HIP EXTENSION FROM ELBOWS

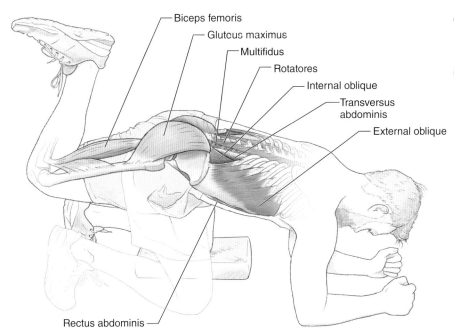

Biceps femoris
Glutcus maximus
Multifidus
Rotatores
Internal oblique
Transversus abdominis
External oblique
Rectus abdominis

(continued)

QUADRUPED HIP EXTENSION FROM ELBOWS *(continued)*

Execution

1. Begin in a quadruped position with your forearms on the ground and elbows aligned under shoulders and knees aligned under the hips. Place one knee on a pad and one knee off the pad.
2. Inhale through the nose before beginning the exercise. Exhale through the mouth as you slowly lift the knee that is not on the pad off the ground until it is parallel with the ground.
3. Extend your hip, reaching your heel toward the ceiling while maintaining a neutral spinal position.
4. Inhale as you return your knee to the start position. Repeat on the opposite side.

Muscles Involved

Primary:

- Rectus abdominis
- Diaphragm
- Internal oblique
- External oblique
- Transversus abdominis
- Multifidus
- Rotatores

Secondary:

- Gluteus maximus
- Biceps femoris

FUNCTIONAL FOCUS

The focus of the quadruped hip extension is to develop dissociation between extension of the hip and extension of the spine and pelvis. Athletes often compensate for lack of hip extension and anti-extension core strength by substituting lumbar extension, putting them at risk for low back pain. During proper execution of this exercise, you should fully extend your hip with no compensatory movement through the lumbar spine.

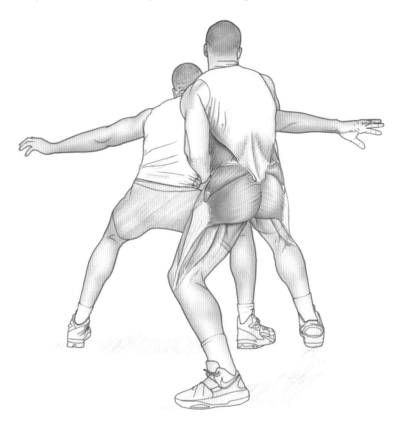

SUPINE BAND HIP FLEXION

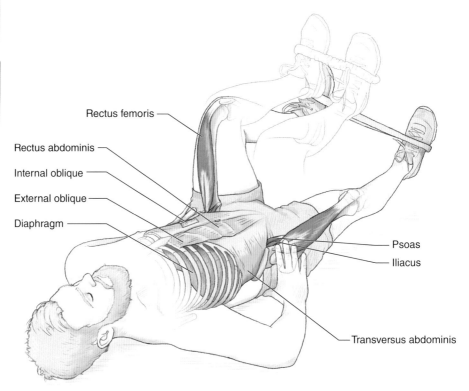

Rectus femoris

Rectus abdominis

Internal oblique

External oblique

Diaphragm

Psoas

Iliacus

Transversus abdominis

Execution

1. Begin lying supine with both knees flexed toward the chest above 90 degrees and a light band looped around the arches of the feet.
2. Inhale through the nose before beginning the exercise. Exhale through the mouth as you slowly extend one leg out straight while maintaining full flexion of the opposing hip, resisting the increased tension in the band.
3. Inhale as you return your knee to the start position. Repeat on the opposite side.

Muscles Involved

Primary:

- Psoas
- Iliacus
- Rectus femoris

Secondary:

- Rectus abdominis
- Diaphragm
- Internal oblique
- External oblique
- Transversus abdominis

(continued)

SUPINE BAND HIP FLEXION *(continued)*

FUNCTIONAL FOCUS

The focus of this drill is to build isolated strength in the hip flexor musculature, specifically the psoas and iliacus muscles, while also developing stability of the pelvis and lumbar spine in the presence of opposing hip flexion and extension. The ability to actively flex and extend the hips using the psoas and iliacus while also controlling pelvic positioning is paramount to efficient running and the prevention of hip flexor strains during sprinting and in sports with frequent cutting and change of direction, such as soccer.

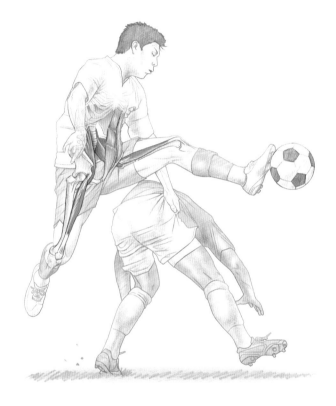

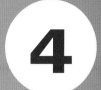

PLYOMETRIC AND MEDICINE BALL EXERCISES

In the vast majority of athletic competitions, the ability to move fast and explosively is paramount to success. The athlete who jumps the highest, runs the fastest, and hits the hardest is more often than not the one who wins the competition. For that reason, power training is a vital piece of the functional training puzzle.

In designing functional training programs, one should be sure to include a variety of power drills for the upper and lower body, done both bilaterally and unilaterally and in all planes of motion. A well-balanced program of power development drills ensures that the athlete properly prepares for the unpredictability of the sporting environment.

In addition to improving performance, plyometric and medicine ball exercises are a fundamental tool for preventing injuries in sport. Progressively exposing athletes to high-velocity movements can train the nervous system to reflexively stabilize more effectively, as well as develop the local tissue resiliency necessary to withstand the demands of high-velocity sports.

JUMP, HOP, AND BOUND

Before proceeding, you should understand some basic terminology as it relates lower-body power drills. Universal terminology is important to ensure clear communication between fellow coaches as well as between coaches and athletes. Although coaches and athletes often use these terms interchangeably, this text adheres to the following definitions:

Jump: Taking off on two legs and landing on two legs

Hop: Taking off on one leg and landing on the same leg

Bound: Taking off on one leg and landing on the opposite leg

It is important to include a variety of lower-body plyometric exercises in your programming. Both bilateral and unilateral drills should have a place in any well-balanced sport performance program. In an effort to ensure your health, focus on challenging your ability to decelerate and produce power in all planes of motion just as you would need to do on the field of play. The dynamic nature of competitive sport requires athletes to decelerate and reaccelerate in the sagittal, frontal, and transverse planes; and by programming jumps, hops, and bounds you can ensure that you are sufficiently prepared for the stressors you will face during competition.

MEDICINE BALL THROWS

Just as jump, hop, and bound variations are effective tools for power development in the lower body, you should include medicine ball drills in your program for power development in the upper body. Throwing low- to moderate-weight medicine balls (2-10 lb [0.9-4.5 kg]) allows for the high-velocity movement and high-threshold motor unit recruitment necessary to develop power in the upper body. Additionally, overhead medicine ball throwing can be especially valuable to condition your shoulder for the eccentric stresses that occur during the deceleration phase of throwing. When selecting medicine ball exercises, you should purposefully choose exercises that develop power in the major patterns represented in sports.

POWER TRAINING FOR THE GENERAL POPULATION

Often coaches and trainees alike assume that power training should be reserved for athletes. However, the general population can benefit greatly from power development training as well. As people age, their nervous system slows down and loses the ability to coordinate powerful high-threshold motor unit contractions. An inability to express lower-body power leads to a reduction in walking speed and a predisposition to tripping and accidental falls. With this in mind, power exercises should be included in programs for the general population and aging adults to maintain neuromuscular efficiency as they age.

DECELERATION BEFORE ACCELERATION

When one thinks about power training, one often thinks of people leaping into the air, but how often does one think about how they land?

Deceleration is an often-overlooked component in the design of programs that develop an efficient, injury-resistant athlete. Thanks to gravity, with every jump, hop, and bound, there is also a landing. As in any high-speed activity, safety has to do with how individuals slow down, not how they speed up. Would you drive fast in a sports car without brakes? Would you jump out of an airplane without a parachute?

It is common to see athletes suffer catastrophic injuries when landing a jump or planting a foot to decelerate and change direction, but athletes are rarely injured when they are concentrically producing force and accelerating. With this in mind, it is imperative for coaches to focus on improving athletes' ability to land and absorb forces eccentrically. Eccentric strength, specifically dynamic eccentric strength, developed in plyometric drills is the musculo-skeletal braking system.

Aside from reducing injuries, the ability to decelerate efficiently allows you to produce more force concentrically after landing. The ability to land in a stable, powerful position will protect your joints and put you in a better position to use elastic energy to explode back upward during the amortization phase of the contraction, in which you transition from the eccentric phase to the concentric phase of the movement.

You can develop eccentric deceleration strength and proper landing mechanics by initially performing stability-focused plyometrics, emphasizing "soft landing" and proper joint positioning. Once you are able to demonstrate the ability to decelerate efficiently, you can begin to progress to jumping higher and developing elasticity through dynamic plyometrics.

Proper landing mechanics during deceleration should ensure the alignment between the foot, tibia, femur, pelvis, and torso to lead to efficient load distribution during landing. In a bilateral landing position, the athlete should land with the feet straight and the patella lined up directly over the forefoot with torso upright and centered over the pelvis (see figure 4.1*a*).

In a unilateral landing position, you should land with the foot, knee, hip, and head all aligned in the frontal plane so that force is efficiently absorbed upward through the skeleton (see figure 4.1b).

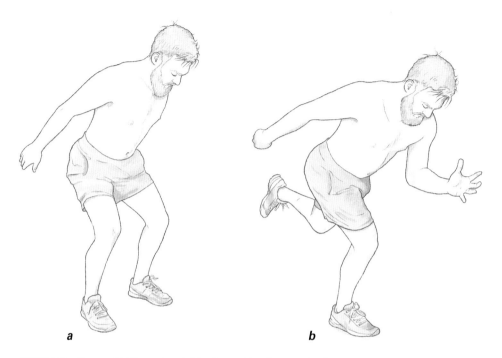

a   b

FIGURE 4.1   Proper (a) bilateral and (b) unilateral landing mechanics.

HURDLE JUMP

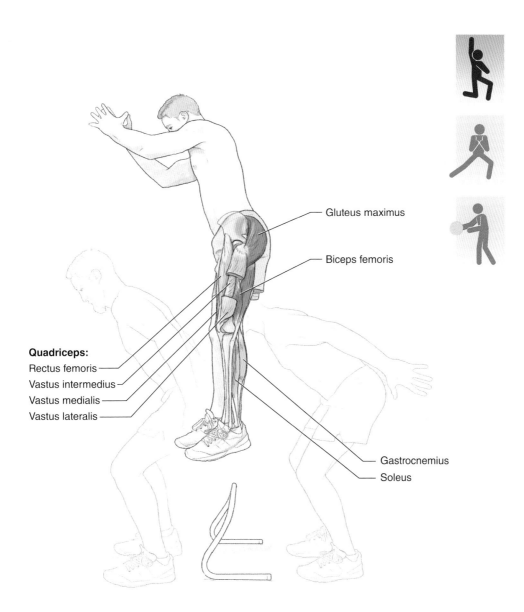

Gluteus maximus

Biceps femoris

Quadriceps:
Rectus femoris
Vastus intermedius
Vastus medialis
Vastus lateralis

Gastrocnemius
Soleus

(continued)

HURDLE JUMP   *(continued)*

Execution

1. Select a set of five hurdles that you can comfortably jump over and arrange them in line, spacing them 3 feet (0.9 m) apart.
2. Stand in an athletic position with your feet parallel, shoulder-width apart, knees bent, and hands next to the hips.
3. Jump over the hurdle by forcefully extending the hips, knees, and ankles and driving your arms up.
4. Land softly on the opposite side of the hurdle in an athletic position with feet shoulder-width apart, knees bent, and feet flat. Hold this position for two seconds. Repeat for the programmed repetitions.

Muscles Involved

Primary:

- Gluteus maximus
- Hamstrings (biceps femoris, semimembranosus, semitendinosus)

Secondary:

- Soleus
- Gastrocnemius
- Quadriceps (rectus femoris, vastus lateralis, vastus medialis, vastus intermedius)

FUNCTIONAL FOCUS

The hurdle jump is a foundational power exercise that should be used to develop bilateral lower-body power and deceleration mechanics. You can use this drill as an introductory jumping progression to build eccentric jumping and landing skills before progressing to unilateral hopping drills.

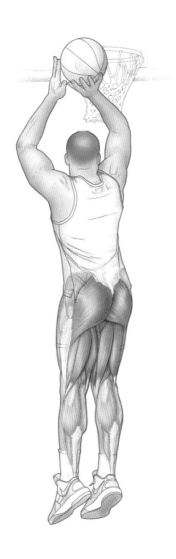

45-DEGREE BOUND

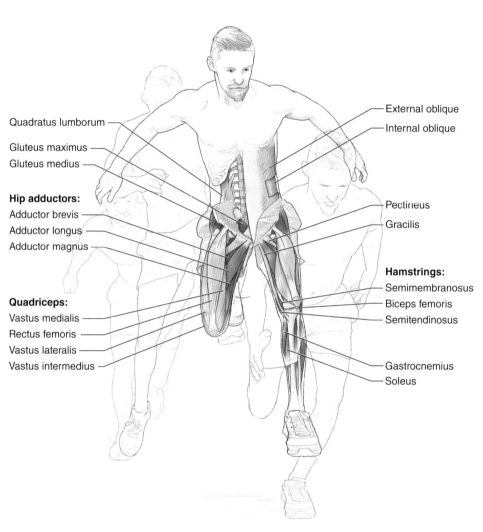

Quadratus lumborum

Gluteus maximus
Gluteus medius

Hip adductors:
Adductor brevis
Adductor longus
Adductor magnus

Quadriceps:
Vastus medialis
Rectus femoris
Vastus lateralis
Vastus intermedius

External oblique
Internal oblique

Pectineus
Gracilis

Hamstrings:
Semimembranosus
Biceps femoris
Semitendinosus

Gastrocnemius
Soleus

Execution

1. Begin in a single-leg athletic position, with one leg off the ground. Center yourself over your support leg by aligning your toes, knee, foot, hip, and head.

2. Bound forward and upward at a 45-degree angle from the midline and land on the opposite leg at a 45-degree angle.

3. Land softly on the opposite leg in the same single-leg athletic position you started in. Hold this position for two seconds after landing. Repeat on the opposite leg.

Muscles Involved

Primary:

- Gluteus maximus
- Gluteus medius
- Hip adductors (adductor longus, adductor magnus, adductor brevis)
- Soleus
- Gastrocnemius
- Hamstrings (semitendinosus, semimembranosus, biceps femoris)

Secondary:

- Quadratus lumborum
- Internal oblique
- External oblique
- Quadriceps (rectus femoris, vastus lateralis, vastus medialis, vastus intermedius)
- Pectineus
- Gracilis

(continued)

45-DEGREE BOUND *(continued)*

VARIATION

Lateral Bound

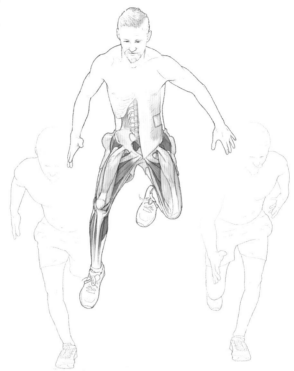

The lateral bound can be used as a regression or an easier version of the 45-degree bound because it requires you to stabilize only in the frontal plane rather than having to decelerate in multiple planes of motion. Begin in a single-leg athletic position with one leg off the ground. Center yourself over your support leg by aligning your toes, knee, foot, hip, and head. Jump laterally and up to land on the opposite leg. Land softly on the opposite leg in the same single-leg athletic position you started in. Hold this position for two seconds after landing. Repeat on the opposite leg.

SINGLE-LEG HURDLE HOP

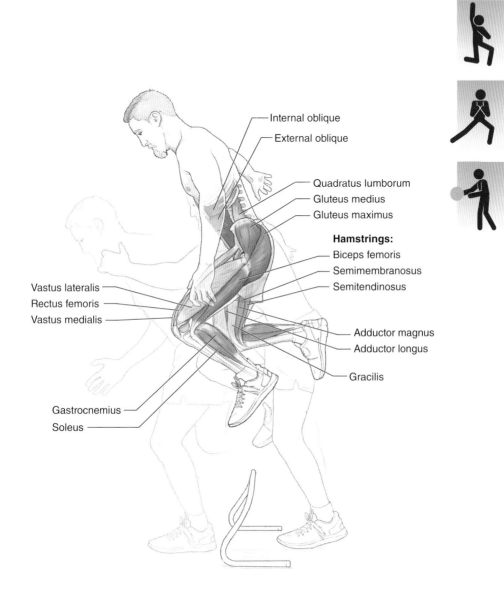

Internal oblique

External oblique

Quadratus lumborum

Gluteus medius

Gluteus maximus

Hamstrings:

Biceps femoris

Semimembranosus

Semitendinosus

Vastus lateralis

Rectus femoris

Vastus medialis

Adductor magnus

Adductor longus

Gracilis

Gastrocnemius

Soleus

(continued)

PLYOMETRIC

SINGLE-LEG HURDLE HOP *(continued)*

Execution

1. Select a set of five hurdles that you can comfortably jump over and arrange them in line, spacing them 3 feet (0.9 m) apart. Stand approximately 1 foot (0.3 m) from the first hurdle in a single-leg position with one leg off the ground. Center yourself over your support leg by aligning your toes, knee, foot, hip, and head.
2. Hop over the hurdle by forcefully extending your hip, knee, and ankle and driving your arms up.
3. Land softly on the same leg on the opposite side of the hurdle in the same athletic position you started in.
4. Hold the landing position for two seconds before moving to the next hurdle. Repeat on the opposite leg.

Muscles Involved

Primary:

- Gluteus maximus
- Gluteus medius
- Hip adductors (adductor longus, adductor magnus, adductor brevis)
- Soleus
- Gastrocnemius
- Hamstrings (semitendinosus, semimembranosus, biceps femoris)

Secondary:

- Quadratus lumborum
- Internal oblique
- External oblique
- Vastus medialis
- Vastus lateralis
- Rectus femoris
- Pectineus
- Gracilis

FUNCTIONAL FOCUS

The single-leg hurdle hop is a unilateral focused lower-body power and deceleration drill. This drill is especially valuable to improve unilateral rate of force production for running and cutting and eccentric landing skills to reduce lower-body, noncontact injuries.

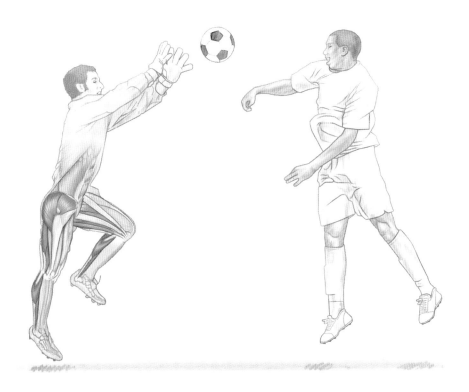

EXPLOSIVE STEP-UPS

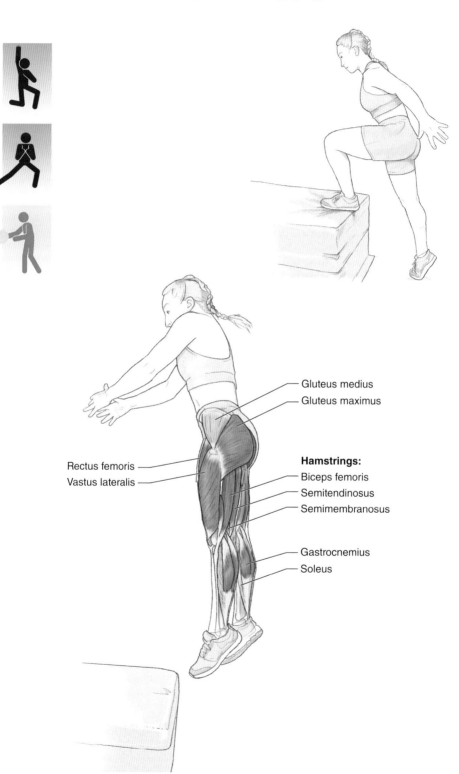

Gluteus medius
Gluteus maximus

Rectus femoris
Vastus lateralis

Hamstrings:
Biceps femoris
Semitendinosus
Semimembranosus

Gastrocnemius
Soleus

Execution

1. Stand 6 inches (15 cm) in front of a 12- to 18-inch (30 to 46 cm) plyometric box or wall of mats with one foot on top and one foot on the ground.
2. Jump straight upward off the foot that is on top of the box, fully extending your knee, hip, and ankle.
3. In midair, switch positions of the legs so that you land with your opposite foot on top of the box.
4. Repeat and continually alternate sides for the programmed repetitions.

Muscles Involved

Primary:

- Gluteus maximus
- Hamstrings (semitendinosus, semimembranosus, biceps femoris)
- Quadriceps (rectus femoris, vastus lateralis, vastus medialis, vastus intermedius)
- Gastrocnemius

Secondary:

- Gluteus medius
- Soleus

(continued)

EXPLOSIVE STEP-UPS *(continued)*

FUNCTIONAL FOCUS

Explosive step-ups are a plyometric drill used to develop the explosive strength necessary for acceleration and the initial push-off for sprinting. The alternating nature of the drill requires a high level of strength and coordination and transfers well to developing sprinting athletes.

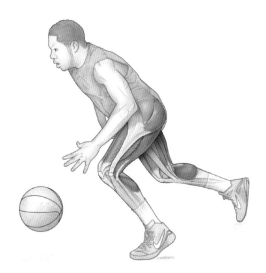

OVERHEAD MEDICINE BALL THROW

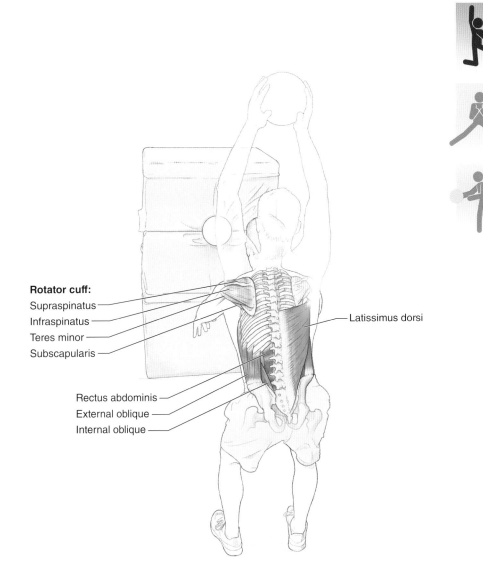

Rotator cuff:
Supraspinatus
Infraspinatus
Teres minor
Subscapularis

Latissimus dorsi

Rectus abdominis
External oblique
Internal oblique

(continued)

OVERHEAD MEDICINE BALL THROW *(continued)*

Execution

1. Stand with your feet shoulder-width apart and raise a 2- to 4-pound (0.9 to 1.8 kg) medicine ball straight overhead. Come onto the balls of the feet, standing as tall as possible.

2. Snap down through the hips and throw the ball as hard and fast as possible at chest height toward the wall.

Muscles Involved

Primary:

- Latissimus dorsi
- Rectus abdominis
- Internal oblique
- External oblique

Secondary:

- Rotator cuff (infraspinatus, supraspinatus, subscapularis, teres minor)

FUNCTIONAL FOCUS

The purpose of the overhead medicine ball throw is to develop integrated anterior core and upper-body throwing power. Throwing the ball as fast as possible develops concentric muscular power through the rectus abdominis and latissimus dorsi while training dynamic eccentric strength through rotator cuff and scapular stabilizing musculature.

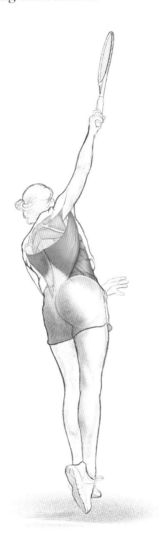

STANDING MEDICINE BALL SIDE TOSS

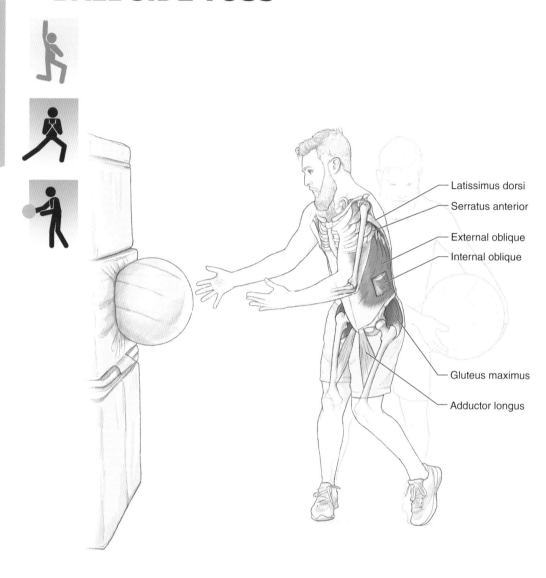

Latissimus dorsi

Serratus anterior

External oblique

Internal oblique

Gluteus maximus

Adductor longus

Execution

1. Stand about 3 feet (0.9 m) from a wall or wall of mats, side to the wall, in an athletic position.
2. Hold a 6- to 10-pound (2.7 to 4.5 kg) medicine ball in your hands in front of your outer hip.
3. Rotate your hips and shoulders toward the wall and forcefully toss the ball at waist height to the wall.
4. Perform the programmed repetitions and repeat on the opposite side.

Muscles Involved

Primary:

- External oblique
- Internal oblique
- Gluteus maximus

Secondary:

- Adductor longus
- Serratus anterior
- Latissimus dorsi

(continued)

STANDING MEDICINE BALL SIDE TOSS *(continued)*

FUNCTIONAL FOCUS

The medicine ball side toss is used to develop full-body power expression in the transverse and frontal planes. This is an effective drill to teach athletes how to produce power and transfer force from their lower extremity to their upper extremity—motions similar to those seen during throwing, swinging, twisting, and punching.

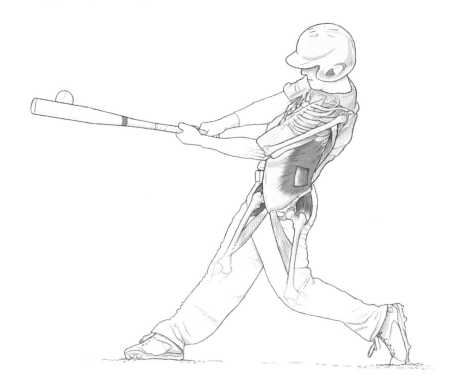

STANDING MEDICINE BALL CHEST PASS

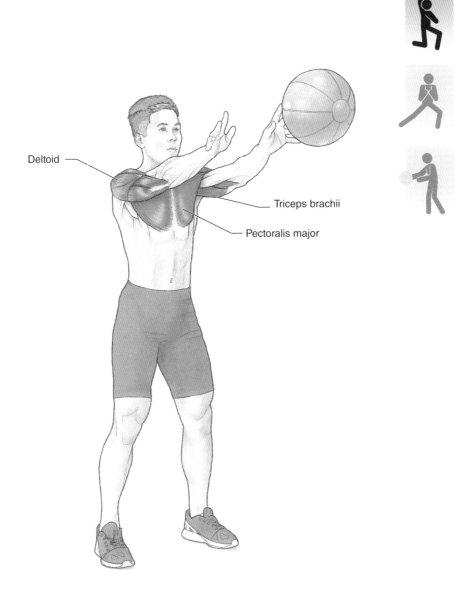

Deltoid

Triceps brachii

Pectoralis major

(continued)

STANDING MEDICINE BALL CHEST PASS   *(continued)*

Execution

1. Stand about 4 feet (1.2 m) from a wall, facing the wall, in an athletic position.
2. Holding the medicine ball at the chest, hip hinge by sitting the hips back away from the wall.
3. Forcefully drive the hips forward and throw the ball straight ahead to the wall.
4. Repeat for the programmed repetitions.

Muscles Involved

Primary:

- Pectoralis major
- Deltoid
- Triceps brachii

Secondary:

- Infraspinatus
- Teres minor

VARIATION

Sprint Start Chest Pass

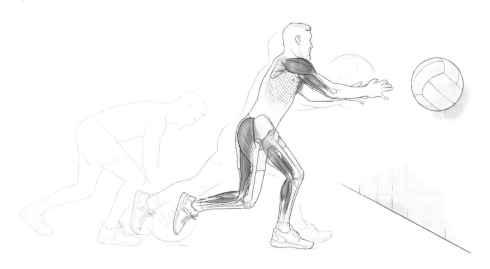

MEDICINE BALL

The sprint start chest pass can be used as a progression, or a more difficult variation, once you have mastered the standing chest pass. This drill develops full-body integrated power, teaching you how to effectively transfer force from the lower body to the upper body into an acceleration sprint pattern.

Stand in a staggered position, feet shoulder-width apart, with the heel of your front foot aligned with the toe of your rear foot. Squat down, placing your hands on the medicine ball in front of you with the majority of your body weight loaded onto your front leg. Forcefully drive your body forward, pushing through the lead leg while simultaneously using your chest and arms to drive the ball forward into the wall.

ROTATIONAL ONE-ARM CHEST PASS

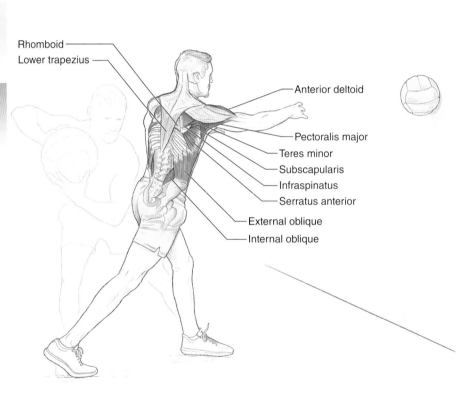

Rhomboid
Lower trapezius
Anterior deltoid
Pectoralis major
Teres minor
Subscapularis
Infraspinatus
Serratus anterior
External oblique
Internal oblique

Execution

1. Stand approximately 6 feet (1.8 m) from the wall in an athletic position with your feet shoulder-width apart, knees bent, and hip flexed. Hold a 4-pound (1.8 kg) medicine ball with both hands in front of your outside shoulder, with your outside elbow raised up high so that your arm is parallel to the floor.
2. Throw the ball at the wall by forcefully rotating your hips and torso and pushing the ball through the palm of the outside hand.
3. Repeat and continually alternate sides for the programmed repetitions.

Muscles Involved

Primary:

- Pectoralis major
- Anterior deltoid
- Serratus anterior
- Rotator cuff (infraspinatus, supraspinatus, subscapularis, teres minor)
- Internal oblique
- External oblique

Secondary:

- Pectoralis minor
- Lower trapezius
- Rhomboids

(continued)

MEDICINE BALL

ROTATIONAL ONE-ARM CHEST PASS *(continued)*

FUNCTIONAL FOCUS

The rotational one-arm chest pass should be programmed to develop upper-body rotational power for throwing and combat sports. This drill teaches you to produce power in the transverse plane and effectively transfer force from the hips through the trunk musculature and into the shoulder and rotator cuff.

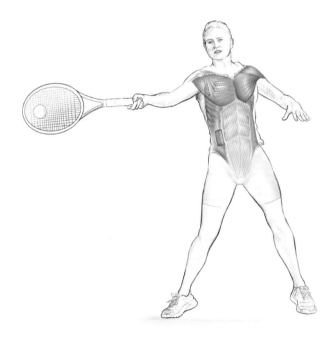

HEAVY IMPLEMENT POWER EXERCISES

5

As a competitive athlete, you should continually search for methods to increase your explosive power. Increased overall power production results in athletes who can run faster, jump higher, and hit harder. You should be performing movements that are heavily loaded and done at high velocity with the goal of improving the firing of the nervous system and the development of fast-twitch, type II muscle fibers.

When learned properly, Olympic lifts like hang cleans and hang snatches, as well as alternatives like kettlebell swings, dumbbell snatches, and sled marching, can be extremely valuable tools to develop explosive power that translates directly to explosive sprinting and jumping in competitive sports.

RATE OF FORCE DEVELOPMENT

The ultimate goal of performing heavy implement power exercises is to improve your rate of force development. You train to move the heaviest load, at the greatest rate of speed that results in the highest power output. Going back to fundamental physics, the equation for power is as follows:

$$\text{Power} = (\text{Force} \times \text{Distance}) / \text{Time}$$

Moving the largest amount of weight the farthest distance, at the fastest rate of speed, will result in the largest power output. It is important to keep this equation in mind when selecting appropriate exercises and weights to ensure you are developing peak power. Power is directly dependent on the variables of load, speed, and distance traveled. While the distance traveled is a fixed variable, dependent on the limb lengths and exercise selection, the load and speed are dependent on weight selection and execution of the exercise.

You should be conscious of how you select load to optimize expression of power during heavy implement power drills. Perform these exercises with the intent of moving the implement at the greatest rate of speed to drive adaptations to the nervous system and muscle fiber quality. With reference to sports, athletes who can produce the most power are often going to be the ones who jump the highest and run the fastest. When it comes specifically to heavy implement power exercises, you should aim to perform the exercises in the middle of the force-velocity curve in figure 5.1.

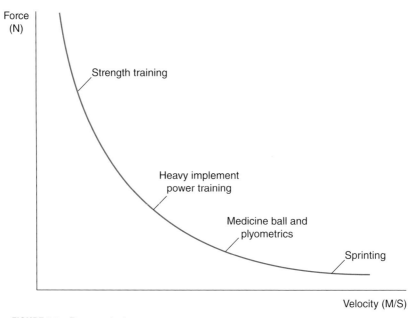

FIGURE 5.1 Force-velocity curve.

With force (load) represented on the Y-axis and velocity (meters/second) represented on the X-axis, you can see plainly how the variables interact to result in differing amounts of power output. The highest levels of force will occur with larger training loads, but at lower speeds. The peak velocity outputs will occur at high speed but with low load. When it comes to generating peak levels of power, you must balance this equation, selecting just the right load that will allow you to produce the absolute highest expression of power. The exercises described in this chapter should be taking place at the apex of this curve, as demonstrated in figure 5.1. Activities like sprinting and plyometrics would occur on the far right side of the curve where speed of movement is greatest, while the strength training exercises covered later in this book would take place on the far left side of the curve where the force production is the greatest.

CENTRAL AND PERIPHERAL ADAPTATIONS TO POWER TRAINING

With the application of power training, you are working to improve coordination between your muscles and nervous system to act in an explosive fashion. Physiologically speaking, you can achieve improvements in power output through two separate pathways. By consistently training explosive power activities, you can improve your efficiency and the output of your central nervous system through an increase in the overall number of motor units recruited, as well as the rate at which they discharge action potentials to the working muscle. These changes to the output of the central nervous system are termed *central adaptations*.

You can also improve your ability to produce power by alternating the ratio of your fast- and slow-twitch muscle fibers; these changes are known as *peripheral adaptations*. All humans have three types of muscle fibers inside the body. These are broken down into type I oxidative, type IIa oxidative-glycolytic, and type IIb adenosine triphosphate (ATP)–glycolytic muscle fibers. These muscle fiber types are separated by their metabolic function and resulting rate of contraction.

Type I oxidative fibers are highly reliant on aerobic metabolism and as a result have a low rate of force development and are highly resistant to fatigue. These fibers would be used primarily during your activities of daily living and for long endurance-based sports like marathon running.

Type IIa oxidative-glycolytic fibers are reliant on both oxidative and glycolytic metabolism; they have a moderately high rate of force production and are resistant to fatigue. Sustained power activities like 400- and 800-meter running or 100- and 200-meter swimming are highly reliant on type IIa muscle fibers.

Type IIb ATP-glycolytic fibers rely on ATP and glycogen stored locally in the muscle. Due to their reliance on local substrate metabolism, they can produce the highest rate of contraction but also fatigue very quickly. Type IIb fibers are the fibers used primarily for short-duration, explosive sprinting and jumping efforts across all sports.

Every individual athlete has a different ratio of muscle fiber dominance depending on genetic inheritance. Some people are born with a higher percentage of type I fibers while others are born with a higher percentage of type II fibers; the former are more favorable for endurance activities, while the latter are more favorable for explosive activities.

Performance coaches want to influence the power expression of the athlete both centrally (central nervous system output) and peripherally (proliferation of type IIb muscle fibers) via training. While both of these variables are highly dependent on genetic inheritance, they can be improved with consistent dedication to heavy implement power training with Olympic lifts, kettlebell swings, dumbbell snatches, and sled sprints.

DEVELOPING PULSING AND BRACING

Power drills also provide a valuable yet extremely overlooked benefit to the competitive athlete, the ability to "pulse" and brace under dynamic load and impact. Highly explosive athletes possess the ability to pulse or contract and subsequently quickly relax their musculature faster than their less explosive counterparts. This is an extremely valuable skill as it relates to sprinting, striking, throwing, and swinging because translating power to a fluid movement outcome depends heavily on the athlete's ability to relax after the initial contraction.

Additionally, the idea of pulsing can be especially valuable for injury reduction. In contact sports the ability to brace for impact and absorb a hit is dependent on the reactivity of the athlete's nervous system to brace the muscle groups to split around the affected body parts. The explosive and rhythmic pulse that occurs during drills like hang cleans, swings, and snatches can train the athlete's nervous system to pulse more effectively.

ALTERNATIVE POWER DEVELOPMENT METHODS

While Olympic lift variations are a hugely beneficial tool to improve power output, they may be contraindicated for a segment of the population due to the particular sport, injury history, or training timeline. If you are dealing with acute or chronic wrist, shoulder, or back issues, Olympic lifts can be problematic because of the potential impact on the affected joints. Similarly, throwing athletes like baseball players should avoid Olympic-style weightlifting due to cumulative stress on the shoulders, elbows, and wrists. Finally, Olympic lifts often require a learning curve to execute correctly. For athletes who have limited training time, it may be more advantageous for coaches to invest their time in power development exercises that can be mastered and implemented more quickly. Alternative power development exercises like kettlebell swings, dumbbell snatches, and sled marching are alternative methods to develop explosive power when Olympic lifts are contraindicated for the athlete.

BARBELL HANG CLEAN

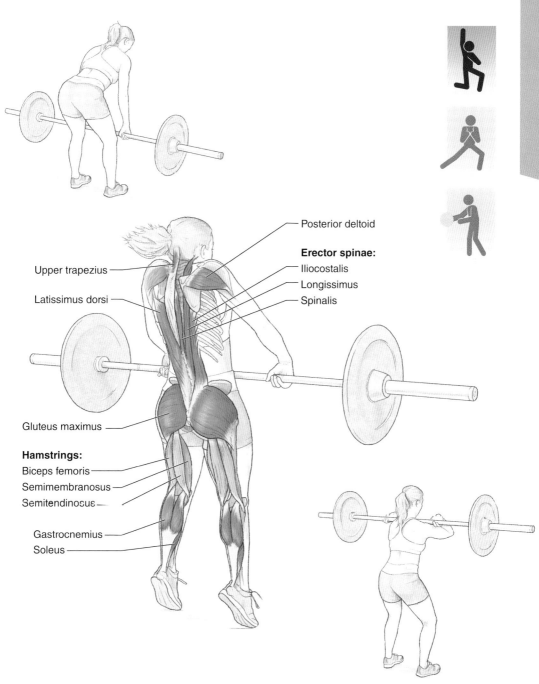

Upper trapezius

Latissimus dorsi

Gluteus maximus

Hamstrings:
Biceps femoris
Semimembranosus
Semitendinosus

Gastrocnemius
Soleus

Posterior deltoid

Erector spinae:
Iliocostalis
Longissimus
Spinalis

(continued)

BARBELL HANG CLEAN   *(continued)*

Execution

1. Stand tall with your feet hip-width apart; hold the bar in front of your hips with your hands slightly outside shoulder width.
2. Pull your shoulders back, curl your wrists, and slightly bend your knees. Slide the bar down your thighs, and hinge your hips backward until the bar is above your knees and your chest is over the bar.
3. Keeping the bar close to your body, jump, shrug, and pull the bar upward. Drive your elbows outward and high toward the ceiling. As the bar reaches chest height, squat under the bar, bringing your elbows forward and finishing the movement in a quarter front squat position.
4. Return the bar to the starting position under control and perform again for the programmed repetitions.

Muscles Involved

Primary:

- Upper trapezius
- Erector spinae (iliocostalis, longissimus, spinalis)
- Latissimus dorsi
- Gluteus maximus
- Soleus
- Gastrocnemius
- Posterior deltoid

Secondary:

- Hamstrings (semitendinosus, semimembranosus, biceps femoris)
- Quadriceps (rectus femoris, vastus lateralis, vastus medialis, vastus intermedius)

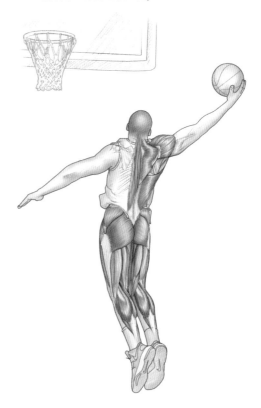

FUNCTIONAL FOCUS

The purpose of including Olympic lifts in the training program is to develop full-body explosive power. The key factor to improving vertical jumping ability is to improve your ability to rapidly produce high levels of vertical force. Barbell hang cleans and snatches train the muscles and movement patterns used for vertical propulsion, making them great exercise choices to improve vertical jump.

VARIATION

Barbell Hang Snatch

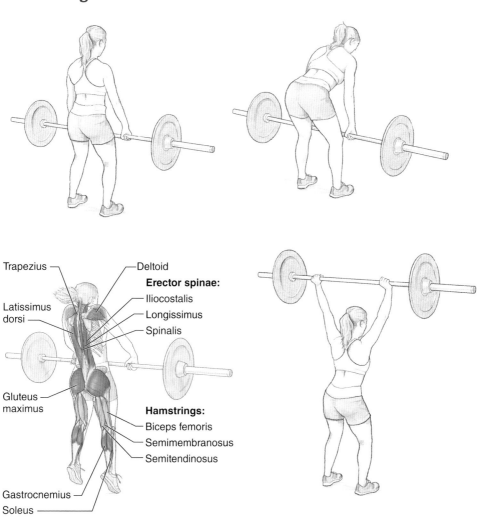

Trapezius
Deltoid
Erector spinae:
Iliocostalis
Latissimus dorsi
Longissimus
Spinalis
Gluteus maximus
Hamstrings:
Biceps femoris
Semimembranosus
Semitendinosus
Gastrocnemius
Soleus

Standing tall with your feet hip-width apart, hold the bar in front of your thighs with your hands at shoulder width. Pull your shoulders back, curl your wrists, and slightly bend your knees. Slide the bar down your thighs and push your hips backward until the bar is above your knees with your chest over the bar. Keeping the bar close to your body, jump, shrug, and propel the bar upward, overhead. Drive your elbows high and finish the movement with the bar in a quarter overhead squat position. Return the bar to the starting position under control and perform again for the programmed repetitions.

KETTLEBELL SWING

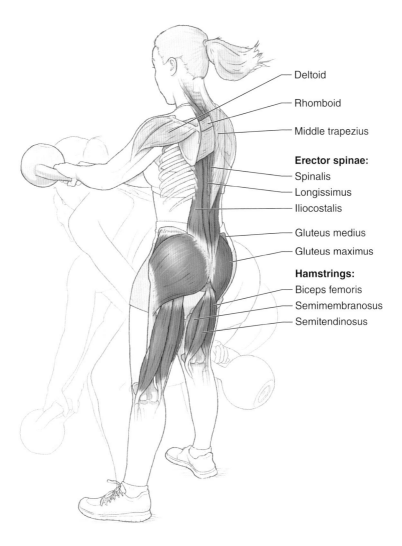

Deltoid

Rhomboid

Middle trapezius

Erector spinae:
Spinalis
Longissimus
Iliocostalis

Gluteus medius
Gluteus maximus

Hamstrings:
Biceps femoris
Semimembranosus
Semitendinosus

Execution

1. Start by standing tall approximately 3 feet (0.9 m) behind a kettlebell. Hip hinge downward, bending your knees and pushing your hips posteriorly. Your shoulders should be positioned on a slight incline above your hips.

2. Reach forward, fully extending your arms, and grab the kettlebell with both hands. Hike the kettlebell backward under your hips toward your glutes while maintaining a strong neutral spine position.

3. Reverse the momentum of the bell by forcefully extending your hips, straightening your knees, and flexing your shoulders upward.

4. Stop the motion when your arms are at chest height and parallel to the ground. Reverse the motion, starting the cycle again, and perform again for the programmed repetitions before returning the kettlebell safely to the ground in front of you.

Muscles Involved

Primary:

- Gluteus maximus
- Gluteus medius
- Hamstrings (semitendinosus, semimembranosus, biceps femoris)
- Erector spinae (iliocostalis, longissimus, spinalis)

Secondary:

- Rhomboids
- Middle trapezius
- Deltoids

(continued)

KETTLEBELL SWING   *(continued)*

FUNCTIONAL FOCUS

The kettlebell swing is a powerful tool to develop explosive hip extension for sports like baseball, tennis, and golf. In all these rotary power sports, athletes are forced to rapidly rotate their pelvis from a position of anterior tilt to a position of posterior tilt before the point of impact in order to create powerful hip extension and translate force from the lower body into the swinging motion. Training heavily loaded kettlebell swings can help you develop explosive power in your hips and pelvis, resulting in a high level of rotational power.

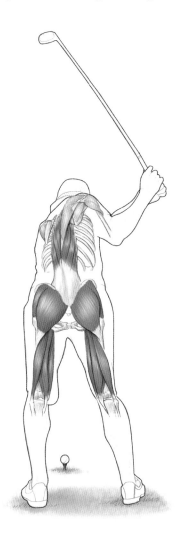

DUMBBELL SNATCH

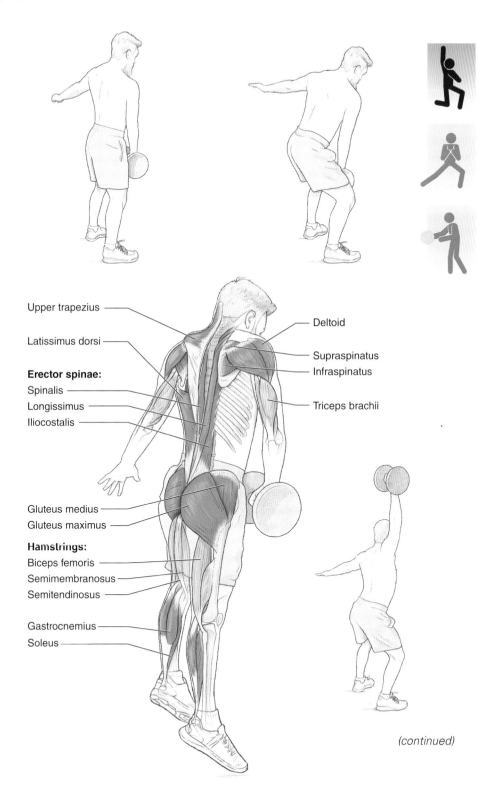

Upper trapezius

Deltoid

Latissimus dorsi

Supraspinatus

Infraspinatus

Erector spinae:
Spinalis
Longissimus
Iliocostalis

Triceps brachii

Gluteus medius
Gluteus maximus

Hamstrings:
Biceps femoris
Semimembranosus
Semitendinosus

Gastrocnemius
Soleus

(continued)

DUMBBELL SNATCH   *(continued)*

Execution

1. Stand in an athletic position with your feet shoulder-width apart and knees slightly bent. Hold a dumbbell in one hand positioned in front of the body, in between the knees, with the hand pronated toward the body.

2. Keeping the dumbbell close to you, jump, shrug, and forcefully propel the dumbbell overhead.

3. Finish with the dumbbell overhead with a straight elbow and wrist. Your lower body should be in roughly a quarter squat.

Muscles Involved

Primary:

- Gluteus medius
- Gluteus maximus
- Erector spinae (iliocostalis, longissimus, spinalis)
- Gastrocnemius
- Soleus
- Deltoid
- Upper trapezius
- Infraspinatus
- Supraspinatus
- Latissimus dorsi

Secondary:

- Triceps brachii
- Hamstrings (semitendinosus, semimembranosus, biceps femoris)

FUNCTIONAL FOCUS

The dumbbell snatch is a valuable tool to develop full-body explosive power with youth athletes or athletes who have a short window of training time. The learning curve for dumbbell snatches is quick, and equipment requirements are low as they call for only the use of a dumbbell. Dumbbell snatches develop full-body power, training the athlete to produce triple extension through the hips, knees, and ankles and transfer that force all the way up to the upper back and shoulder when propelling the dumbbell overhead. An added benefit of the dumbbell snatch is the dynamic stability it develops in the shoulder girdle musculature when forced to decelerate the dumbbell at the end of the movement.

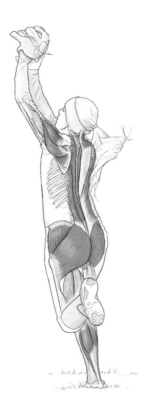

SLED MARCH

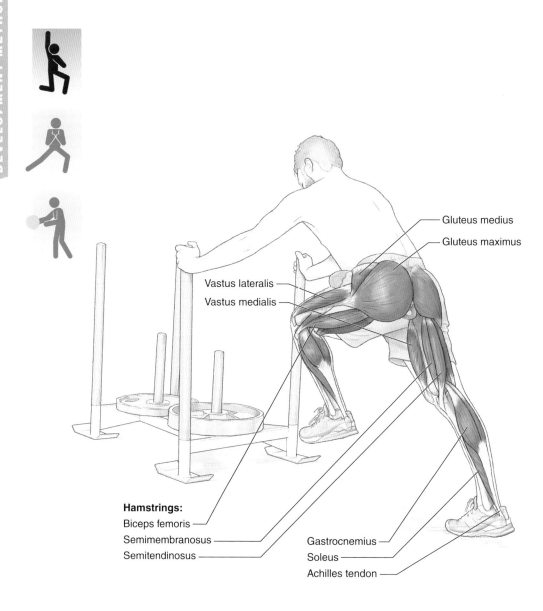

Gluteus medius

Gluteus maximus

Vastus lateralis

Vastus medialis

Hamstrings:
Biceps femoris
Semimembranosus
Semitendinosus

Gastrocnemius
Soleus
Achilles tendon

Execution

1. Load a drive sled with a weight that will allow you to comfortably push in a steady continuous motion. Lean against the drive sled with your hands on the top of the handles, arms straight, and body at a 45-degree angle.

2. Move the sled by marching forward, driving the knees up past the hips and striking your foot to the ground behind your center of mass. Maintain active dorsiflexion of your ankle and maintain a continuous marching rhythm until reaching the programmed distance.

Muscles Involved

Primary:

- Gluteus maximus
- Gluteus medius
- Rectus femoris
- Vastus medialis
- Vastus lateralis
- Hamstrings (semitendinosus, semimembranosus, biceps femoris)
- Gastrocnemius
- Soleus

Secondary:

- Adductor magnus
- Flexor hallucis brevis
- Flexor digitorum brevis
- Achilles tendon

ALTERNATIVE POWER DEVELOPMENT METHODS

(continued)

SLED MARCH *(continued)*

FUNCTIONAL FOCUS

The acceleration phase of sprinting is a dynamic piston-like action that requires the athlete to translate force from the hips to the hamstrings all the way through the lower leg and foot. While traditional weight room exercises can develop general strength and power, the pattern specificity of the sled march exercise provides high levels of carryover to sprint performance on the field of play. Acceleration depends largely on power hip extension from the glutes and hamstrings and plantar flexion from the gastrocnemius and soleus, all of which are stressed directly during the sled march exercise.

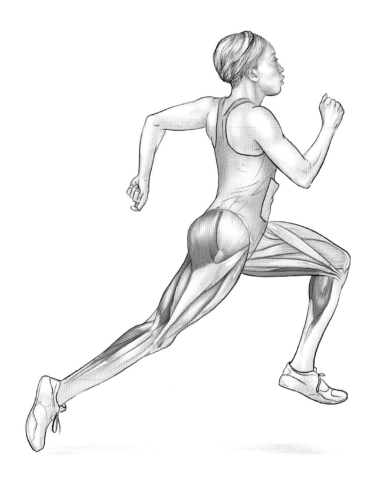

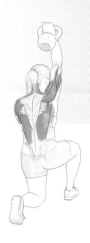

6

UPPER-BODY STRENGTH EXERCISES

The development of upper-body strength, specifically in the muscles surrounding the shoulder girdle, is extremely important for performance enhancement and injury reduction in sports. In traditional bodybuilding-style training, hypertrophy and single-joint exercises are overemphasized for the sake of aesthetic development. While this approach is appropriate for the pursuit of bodybuilding, it does not translate well to functional athletic performance.

When designing functional strength training programs for the development of upper-body strength and power, one should take into account the function of all the muscles articulating from the thorax to the glenohumeral and scapulothoracic joints. The extreme amounts of mobility afforded by the design of the shoulder complex require intricate coactivation of all the surrounding musculature to a safe, efficient, and coordinated outcome during dynamic upper-body movements like throwing, striking, swinging, pushing, and pulling. The rotator cuff muscle group (infraspinatus, supraspinatus, subscapularis, teres minor) and the scapulothoracic stabilizers shown in figure 6.1 are vital to stabilizing the humerus and scapula during sporting activities.

Almost all competitive sports require a huge variety of dynamic movements that stress the anatomy of the upper body. Swinging a tennis racket, pitching a baseball, tackling an opponent, and bracing for impact all require extreme amounts of mobility and stability at the glenohumeral and scapulothoracic joints.

The act of pitching a baseball may require the humerus to rotate with an angular velocity of up to 7,500 degrees per second while accessing extreme amounts of external rotation. To effectively decelerate the shoulder after throwing requires the development of large amounts of eccentric strength in the posterior shoulder musculature, specifically in the latissimus dorsi, infraspinatus, teres minor, rhomboids, and lower trapezius (see figure 6.1). Pulling exercises like the dumbbell row discussed later in this chapter can be

especially effective at developing the posterior stabilizing musculature necessary to complete the throwing motion and protect the health of the shoulder.

The ability to forcefully swing a racket in tennis or strike an opponent with
a punch requires large amounts of strength in scapula protractors as well as
in flexors and abductors of the humerus. Exercises like push-ups and the
incline dumbbell bench press discussed later in this chapter can be especially
valuable in developing the serratus anterior, anterior deltoids, pectoralis major,
and triceps brachii for striking and swinging.

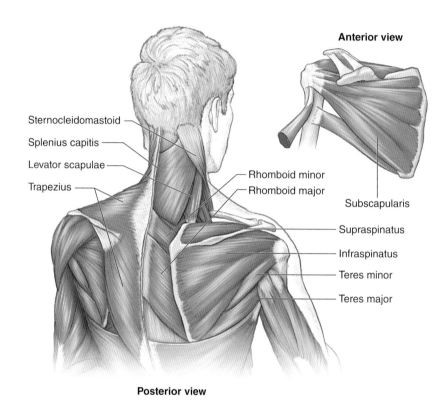

FIGURE 6.1   The muscles of the rotator cuff and the scapular stabilizing musculature.
Development of these muscles is vital for shoulder health and performance in throwing
and contact sport athletes.

PROGRAMMING FOR SHOULDER HEALTH

Due to the influence of bodybuilding and power lifting, many traditional programs place great emphasis on pressing exercises like push-ups and bench press and less emphasis on pulling exercises like chin-ups and rows. This is a mistake that will leave athletes at risk for upper-body injuries. A balanced functional training program should develop all the muscles surrounding the shoulder by devoting equal time to vertical and horizontal pushing and pulling exercises.

To ensure balanced programming, one can break down the upper-body strength exercises into four major categories.

1. **Horizontal push:** Push-up, barbell bench press, incline dumbbell bench press
2. **Vertical push:** Half-kneeling alternating kettlebell overhead press
3. **Horizontal pull:** Dumbbell row
4. **Vertical pull:** Chin-up, pull-up

PUSH-UP

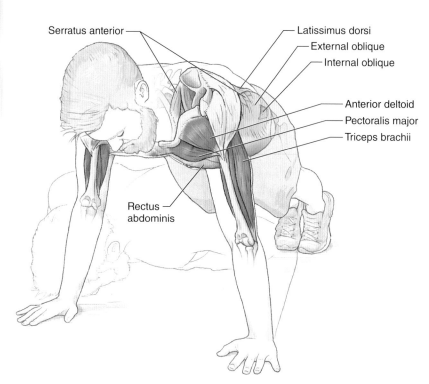

Serratus anterior

Latissimus dorsi

External oblique

Internal oblique

Anterior deltoid

Pectoralis major

Triceps brachii

Rectus abdominis

Execution

1. Begin at the top of a supported, prone push-up position with your legs together and hands just outside shoulder width. Maintain a straight alignment between your head, thoracic spine, and sacrum.

2. Slowly lower yourself under control toward the ground until you are approximately 3 inches (7.6 cm) from the ground. In the bottom position, the humerus should be abducted approximately 45 degrees from the midline of the body.

3. Drive up from the ground forcefully while maintaining straight alignment through the torso. Lock out arms fully at the top of the movement and repeat for the programmed number of repetitions.

Muscles Involved

Primary:

- Pectoralis major
- Triceps brachii
- Anterior deltoid

Secondary:

- Infraspinatus
- Teres minor
- Latissimus dorsi
- Serratus anterior
- Rectus abdominis
- Internal and external obliques

(continued)

PUSH-UP *(continued)*

FUNCTIONAL FOCUS

The push-up directly targets the muscles used to generate power during swinging, striking, and throwing. The closed chain nature of the push-up allows for free movement of the scapula that is not afforded by exercises like barbell bench press in which the scapula is pinned against a bench. Allowing for this natural movement permits development of the glenohumeral and scapular stabilizers like the serratus anterior, infraspinatus, and teres minor in addition to prime movers like the pectoralis major, anterior deltoids, latissimus dorsi, and triceps brachii.

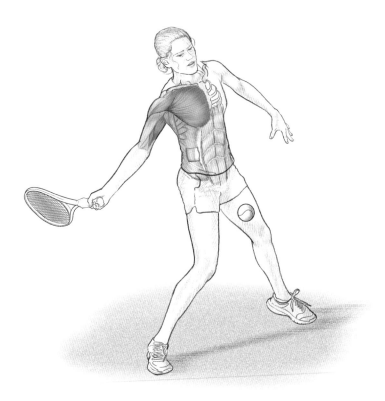

HALF-KNEELING ALTERNATING KETTLEBELL OVERHEAD PRESS

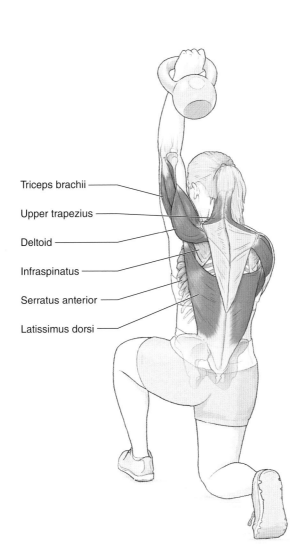

Triceps brachii

Upper trapezius

Deltoid

Infraspinatus

Serratus anterior

Latissimus dorsi

(continued)

HALF-KNEELING ALTERNATING KETTLEBELL OVERHEAD PRESS   *(continued)*

Execution

1. Begin in a half-kneeling position, with the rear ankle dorsiflexed and kettlebells in a front rack position in front of the chest.

2. Maintaining a stable torso, press one arm up overhead, locking it out completely at the top position.

3. Slowly lower the kettlebell down to the start position and repeat the motion with the opposite arm. Continue alternating sides until you complete all the programmed repetitions. Alternate kneeling stance on each subsequent set.

Muscles Involved

Primary:

- Deltoid
- Upper trapezius
- Triceps brachii
- Latissimus dorsi

Secondary:

- Infraspinatus
- Subscapularis
- Serratus anterior

FUNCTIONAL FOCUS

The half-kneeling alternating kettlebell overhead press develops the anterior deltoids and triceps brachii as well as the latissimus dorsi, upper trapezius, infraspinatus, and subscapularis. These muscles are especially important to vertical force production, in sports like basketball and volleyball where the ball is often being shot or served or set overhead. Developing these muscles in the overhead position will not only develop strength specific to the sporting activity but will also improve glenohumeral stability in the overhead position.

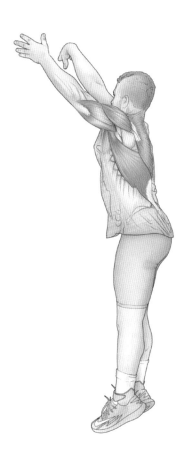

BARBELL BENCH PRESS

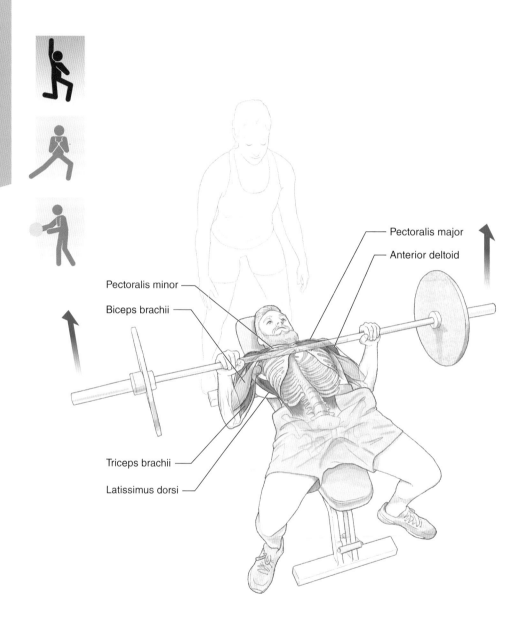

Pectoralis major

Anterior deltoid

Pectoralis minor

Biceps brachii

Triceps brachii

Latissimus dorsi

Execution

1. Begin by lying supine on a bench with your feet firmly planted on the floor. Grab the barbell slightly outside of shoulder width and bring it out of the rack so that it is directly over your shoulder.

2. Create tension in the shoulder girdle by actively externally rotating at the shoulders while firmly gripping the bar. Slowly lower the bar down until it contacts the highest point of your chest.

3. Forcefully, drive the barbell back up, locking out the arms completely at the top. Repeat for the programmed repetitions before returning the barbell to the rack.

Muscles Involved

Primary:

- Pectoralis major
- Anterior deltoid
- Triceps brachii
- Latissimus dorsi

Secondary:

- Pectoralis minor
- Biceps brachii

(continued)

BARBELL BENCH PRESS *(continued)*

FUNCTIONAL FOCUS

The bench press is an effective tool to create hypertrophy of the upper body, which helps to armor the body for collision sports like hockey and football. Additionally, the bench press trains the muscles used to initiate contact in collision sports. Checking another player into the boards or blocking an opponent at the line of scrimmage requires large amounts of strength in the pectoral, deltoid, and triceps muscle groups.

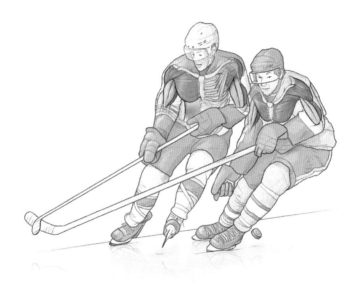

INCLINE DUMBBELL BENCH PRESS

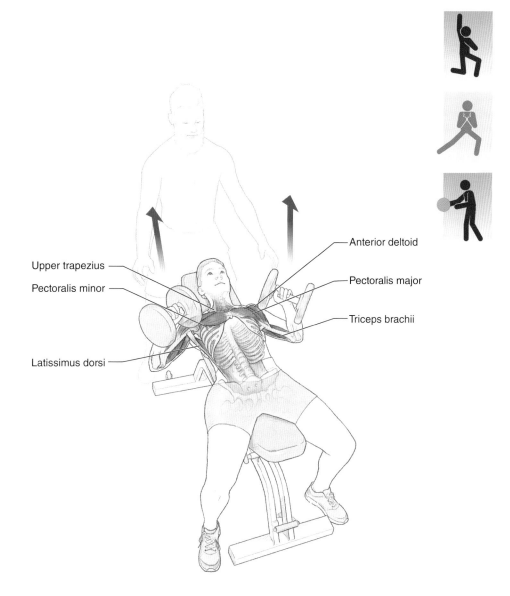

Upper trapezius

Pectoralis minor

Latissimus dorsi

Anterior deltoid

Pectoralis major

Triceps brachii

(continued)

INCLINE DUMBBELL BENCH PRESS   *(continued)*

Execution

1. Begin by lying on an incline bench at approximately a 20-degree incline. Keep your feet firmly planted on the ground throughout the exercise. Bring the dumbbells overhead so they are directly above your shoulders with your elbows straight.

2. Lower the dumbbells downward until they are outside the shoulders and approximately 6 inches (15 cm) above your chest. Drive the dumbbells upward until your arms are locked out.

3. Be sure that your hips stay on the bench and your feet stay on the ground throughout the entire exercise.

Muscles Involved

Primary:

- Anterior deltoid
- Pectoralis major
- Triceps brachii

Secondary:

- Pectoralis minor
- Latissimus dorsi
- Upper trapezius

FUNCTIONAL FOCUS

The incline dumbbell bench press should be programmed to develop strength and power in the upper chest, shoulders, and arms. Strength developed in these areas will translate well to producing power in contact sports like hockey, football, lacrosse, basketball, and boxing. The ability to powerfully strike an opponent while checking or blocking greatly depends on an athlete's upper-body strength development.

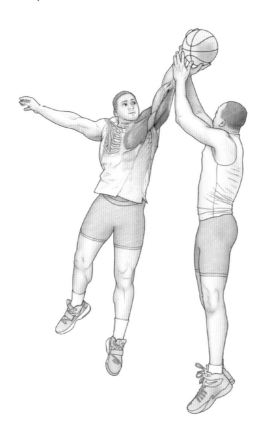

CHIN-UP

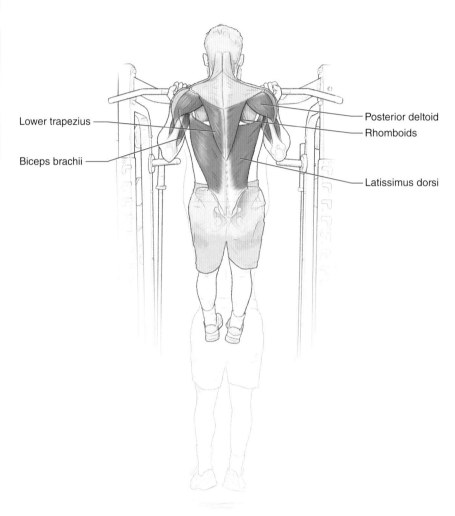

Lower trapezius

Biceps brachii

Posterior deltoid

Rhomboids

Latissimus dorsi

Execution

1. Start in a full hanging position from the bar with your palms supinated, shoulders fully flexed overhead, and elbows fully extended.

2. Forcefully pull your collarbone up to the bar, maintaining a straight alignment from your head to your feet with no jerking or kipping of the torso.

3. Slowly lower yourself downward to the start position until your arms are fully extended. Repeat for the programmed repetitions.

Muscles Involved

Primary:

- Latissimus dorsi
- Biceps brachii
- Rhomboids
- Posterior deltoid
- Lower trapezius

Secondary:

- Rectus abdominis
- Brachialis
- Brachioradialis
- Pronator teres
- Flexor carpi radialis
- Flexor digitorum superficialis

(continued)

CHIN-UP *(continued)*

VARIATION

Pull-Up

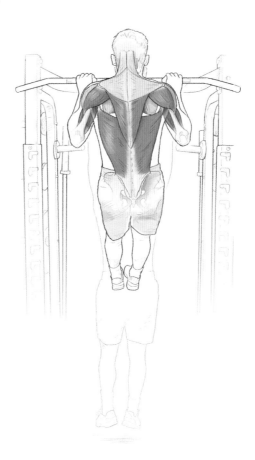

Start in a full hanging position from the bar with the palms pronated and hands just outside shoulder width, shoulders fully flexed overhead, and elbows fully extended. Forcefully pull your collarbone up to the bar, maintaining a straight alignment from your head to your feet with no jerking or kipping of the torso. Slowly lower yourself downward to the start position until your arms are fully extended. Repeat for the programmed repetitions.

DUMBBELL ROW

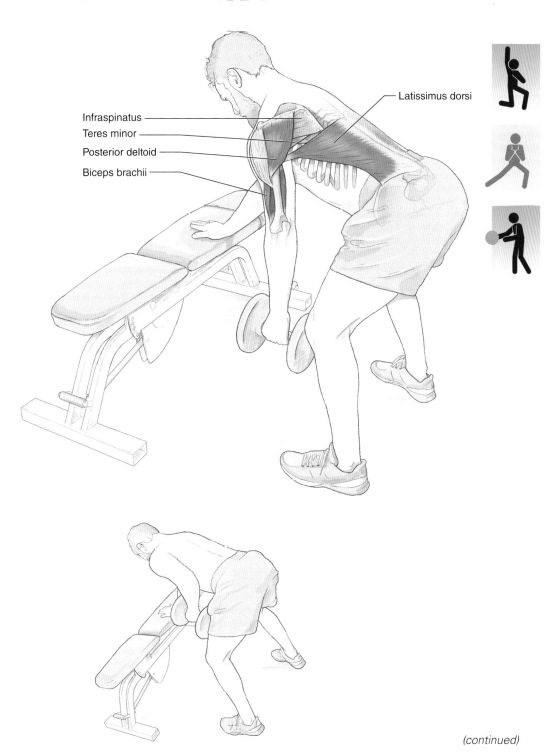

Latissimus dorsi

Infraspinatus

Teres minor

Posterior deltoid

Biceps brachii

(continued)

DUMBBELL ROW   *(continued)*

Execution

1. Begin standing approximately 3 feet (0.9 m) away from a bench with your feet slightly outside shoulder-width apart, knees slightly bent. Hinge at the hips, placing one hand firmly on the bench while maintaining a flat back.

2. Using the opposite arm, grab a dumbbell and row it upward toward the body until it reaches the outside of the rib cage.

3. Slowly lower the dumbbell back down toward the start position without losing your spinal position.

Muscles Involved

Primary:

- Latissimus dorsi
- Posterior deltoid
- Biceps brachii

Secondary:

- Teres minor
- Infraspinatus
- Brachioradialis

FUNCTIONAL FOCUS

The dumbbell row develops the posterior shoulder, upper and middle back musculature (specifically the posterior deltoids), latissimus dorsi, rhomboids, and to a smaller degree the biceps and rotator cuff muscles. These muscles provide stability to the shoulder girdle and scapular complex, protecting the shoulder against instability and providing a strong foundation for pressing or bracing against contact. The muscles of the back and posterior shoulder are integral to the deceleration of the humerus and scapula joint during throwing and overhead striking, and they help to protect the integrity of the gleno-humeral joint capsule and rotator cuff musculature.

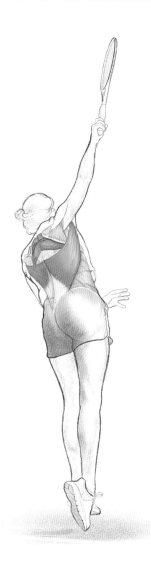

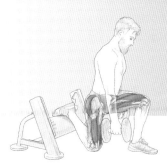

LOWER-BODY STRENGTH EXERCISES

Without question the most valuable asset gained in the weight room to improve performance and reduce injuries in competitive athletics is lower-body strength. Full-body force production always starts in the legs. Whether in sprinting past an opponent, leaping for a lay-up, or swinging a bat, force must be generated by pushing into the ground and then translated throughout the rest of the body. There is no athletic endeavor on this planet that won't benefit from developing lower-body strength.

A simple physics equation represents the ability of an athlete to run fast and jump high. The more force athletes are able to put into the ground, the farther and faster they will be able to move. See the following formula:

$$Force = Mass \times Acceleration$$

The ability of athletes to strike the ground forcefully and accelerate their body mass vertically or horizontally depends greatly on their lower-body strength. It is known that in almost all competitive sports, speed is the ultimate advantage, so lower-body strength training should be prioritized in a functional strength training program.

Even endurance events like distance running can benefit greatly from the inclusion of lower-body strength training. Research has demonstrated that lower-body strength training can markedly improve running economy and reduce the likelihood of running-related injuries like osteoarthritis, plantar fasciitis, stress fractures, and hamstring strains.

HIP-DOMINANT VERSUS KNEE-DOMINANT MOVEMENTS

When designing functional training programs, it is helpful to categorize lower-body strength exercises into either hip-dominant or knee-dominant movements. Organizing all lower-body movements into either of these two subdivisions can ensure simple and balanced programming.

Knee-dominant exercises like goblet squats, split squat variations, and single-leg squats primarily develop the anterior knee extensor musculature like the rectus femoris, vastus medialis, and vastus lateralis while developing the glutes and hamstrings to a lesser degree.

Hip-dominant exercises like deadlifts and bridges focus primarily on development of the posterior chain musculature, specifically the glute and hamstring muscle groups.

BILATERAL VERSUS UNILATERAL LOWER-BODY TRAINING

Beyond categorizing lower-body strength exercises into hip-dominant and knee-dominant movements, one can further divide them into bilateral and unilateral movements. Traditional bodybuilding- and powerlifting-focused training approaches have placed heavy emphasis on bilateral movements like back squats and straight bar deadlifts for the development of muscular strength and hypertrophy. While these approaches may have high levels of carryover for sports like competitive powerlifting, they have much less carryover to more athletic endeavors that involve running, jumping, and rapid change of direction. Bilateral lower-body strength exercises do still have a place in a complete functional training program, especially for beginners. Goblet squats are a great entry-level strength training exercise to begin developing foundational lower-body strength, and trap bar deadlifts are a valuable tool to develop posterior chain strength and hypertrophy.

LOWER-BODY FUNCTIONAL STRENGTH TRAINING IS UNILATERAL

When constructing a functional training program, one should look to include exercises that challenge the body in a way that is similar to the way it will be challenged in sport. Structurally and neurologically, human beings are unilaterally dominant creatures, designed to move in contralateral patterns with one limb at a time. Choosing training strategies that are congruent with how human bodies are designed will yield more effective and efficient programming.

Keeping this in mind, it is important to ensure that unilateral lower-body exercises make up the majority of any lower-body strength training program due to their high level of carryover to the demands of sport, as well as their tendency to spare the spine from excess loading. Competitive sports are played primarily on one leg at a time, and training approaches should reflect those demands to ensure maximal carryover to sporting activities. The functional demands of the lower-body musculature completely change when you go from a bilateral stance to a unilateral stance. While you stand on two legs, the balanced nature of your stance does not require high levels of activity in the frontal and transverse plane stabilizing musculature. Conversely, the instant you remove one leg from the ground, your body is forced to recruit a number of medial and lateral stabilizer muscles in order to maintain alignment in the frontal and transverse planes. The medial and lateral abdominal, hip, and lower-leg muscles must work in coactivation to maintain positioning of the trunk, pelvis, femur, and lower leg in single-leg stance.

It is clear why unilateral training is so important for injury reduction in competitive athletics. Using unilateral exercises like single-leg squats and deadlifts to develop control of the pelvis, femur, tibia, and foot in a single-leg stance will help you protect the often-injured ligaments and tendons of the knee and ankle.

GOBLET SQUAT

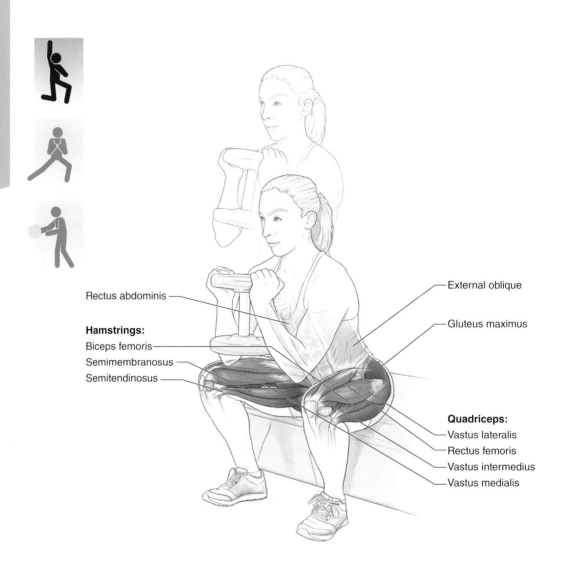

Rectus abdominis

Hamstrings:
Biceps femoris
Semimembranosus
Semitendinosus

External oblique

Gluteus maximus

Quadriceps:
Vastus lateralis
Rectus femoris
Vastus intermedius
Vastus medialis

Execution

1. Begin standing with your feet slightly outside of shoulder width and toes straight ahead. Hold a dumbbell or kettlebell tight against your chest, keeping your elbows pinned tight to the body.

2. Brace for the squat by drawing your ribs downward, slightly posteriorly tilting your pelvis, and creating tension in your hip by actively trying to screw your feet into the floor through external rotation.

3. Lower yourself down under control letting your knees come forward until your femur is at least parallel to the floor. Reverse the motion, driving upward, keeping your chest up and your back flat.

4. Repeat for the programmed repetitions.

Muscles Involved

Primary:

- Quadriceps (rectus femoris, vastus lateralis, vastus medialis, vastus intermedius)
- Gluteus maximus
- Hamstrings (semitendinosus, semimembranosus, biceps femoris)

Secondary:

- Rectus abdominis
- External oblique

(continued)

GOBLET SQUAT *(continued)*

FUNCTIONAL FOCUS

The goblet squat should be the primary exercise choice for developing bilateral knee-dominant strength. This variation of the squat is much easier to learn and carries a much lower injury risk than the traditional back squat. Holding the dumbbell at the chest allows the athlete to maintain a vertical torso and also helps to develop core strength in the rectus abdominis and external obliques, in addition to stressing the quadriceps, glutes, and hamstrings. Developing bilateral knee-dominant strength translates well to bilateral actions like jumping and serves as a foundation to begin developing unilateral strength for beginners or athletes returning from injury.

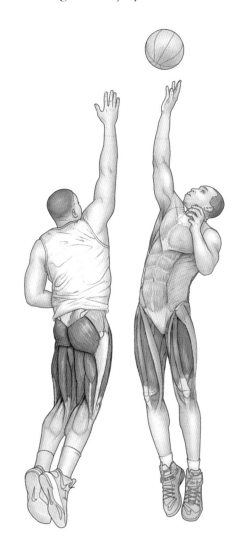

REAR FOOT ELEVATED SPLIT SQUAT

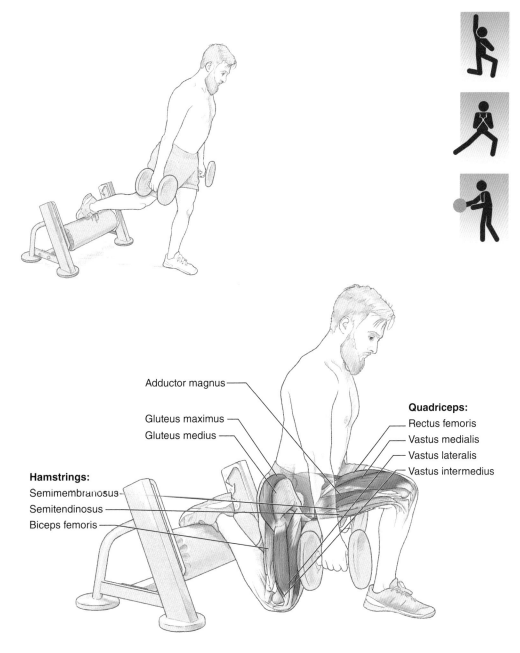

Adductor magnus

Gluteus maximus
Gluteus medius

Quadriceps:
Rectus femoris
Vastus medialis
Vastus lateralis
Vastus intermedius

Hamstrings:
Semimembranosus
Semitendinosus
Biceps femoris

(continued)

REAR FOOT ELEVATED SPLIT SQUAT *(continued)*

Execution

1. Holding dumbbells in each hand, stand with your feet together with a bench or split squat stand positioned perpendicular, approximately 2 feet (0.6 m) behind you. Reach one leg back and position the top side of your foot on the bench or stand.

2. Keeping your chest up tall, lower yourself downward to the ground under control with your lead leg. Maintain alignment of your lead knee in front of the hip and over the top of the foot.

3. Tap your knee on the ground at the bottom of the movement, before forcefully propelling yourself upward to the starting position. Repeat for the programmed repetitions.

Muscles Involved

Primary:

- Quadriceps (rectus femoris, vastus lateralis, vastus medialis, vastus intermedius)
- Gluteus maximus
- Adductor magnus

Secondary:

- Hamstrings (semitendinosus, semimembranosus, biceps femoris)
- Gluteus medius

FUNCTIONAL FOCUS

The use of heavily loaded unilateral knee-dominant exercises like rear foot elevated split squats should be the primary approach to develop functional lower-body strength for athletic performance. Sprinting, hopping, decelerating, and changing directions all rely heavily on functional unilateral strength that cannot be developed with traditional bilateral exercises. Additionally, unilateral exercises loaded with dumbbells rather than bilateral exercises loaded on the spine with a barbell may have a sparing effect on the spine of the athlete, reducing the likelihood of spinal injury.

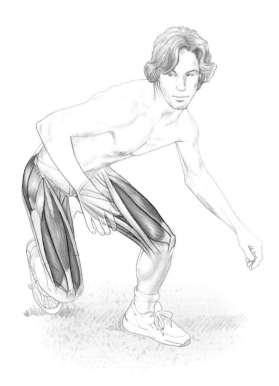

VARIATION

Two-Dumbbell Loaded Split Squat

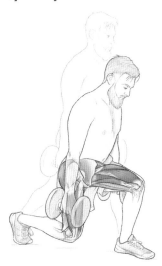

Begin in a half-kneeling position with your right knee down and your left foot in front. The right knee should be directly below the right hip, and the left knee should be directly over the left midfoot. Hold a dumbbell in each hand beside you. Drive the left heel into the ground, driving yourself upward until the left leg is almost full extended. Return to the bottom position, lightly tapping your knee on the ground before repeating the exercise. Repeat for the programmed repetitions. Repeat on the opposite side.

The split squat is a regression from the rear foot elevated split squat that distributes the athlete's weight more evenly between the two legs. The decreased load on the front legs makes this drill easier for beginner trainees who may not have developed adequate strength or who struggle with balance when executing the rear foot elevated split squat.

SINGLE-LEG SQUAT

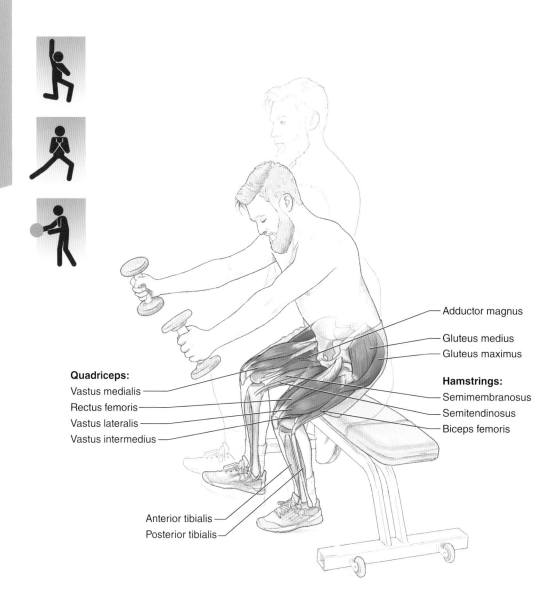

Adductor magnus

Gluteus medius

Gluteus maximus

Quadriceps:

Vastus medialis

Rectus femoris

Vastus lateralis

Vastus intermedius

Hamstrings:

Semimembranosus

Semitendinosus

Biceps femoris

Anterior tibialis

Posterior tibialis

Execution

1. Stand in front of a weight bench or 18-inch (46 cm) box with a 5-pound (7.3 kg) dumbbell in each hand.

2. Reach the weights forward and upward while picking one foot up off the floor and slowly squatting down and toward the bench.

3. Lightly tap your butt on the bench at the bottom, but avoid bouncing and return to the top position. Focus on maintaining alignment between the hip, knee, and foot throughout the entire movement.

4. Perform for the programmed repetitions and repeat on the opposite side.

Muscles Involved

Primary:

- Quadriceps (rectus femoris, vastus lateralis, vastus medialis, vastus intermedius)
- Gluteus maximus
- Gluteus medius
- Adductor magnus

Secondary:

- Hamstrings (semitendinosus, semimembranosus, biceps femoris)
- Anterior tibialis
- Posterior tibialis

(continued)

SINGLE-LEG SQUAT *(continued)*

FUNCTIONAL FOCUS

Multiplanar single-leg strength and stability is fundamental to sport performance and injury reduction. On the field of play, the athlete is constantly stabilizing the foot, ankle, tibia, femur, and pelvis against variable forces in all directions. The single-leg squat provides the closest representation possible in the weight room to mimic the stressors experienced in the lower body on the field of play. When you plant a foot in single-leg stance, the lateral glute musculature, hamstrings, adductors, and quadriceps will all be forced to cocontract to create stability of the femur, just as they are during the single-leg squat exercise. Developing strength and control in the single-leg squat will directly correlate to increased protection from lower-body injuries like anterior cruciate ligament ruptures.

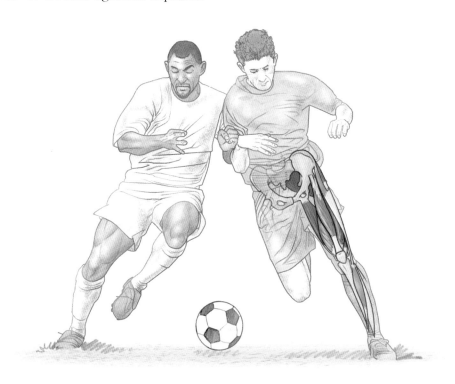

GOBLET LOADED LATERAL SQUAT

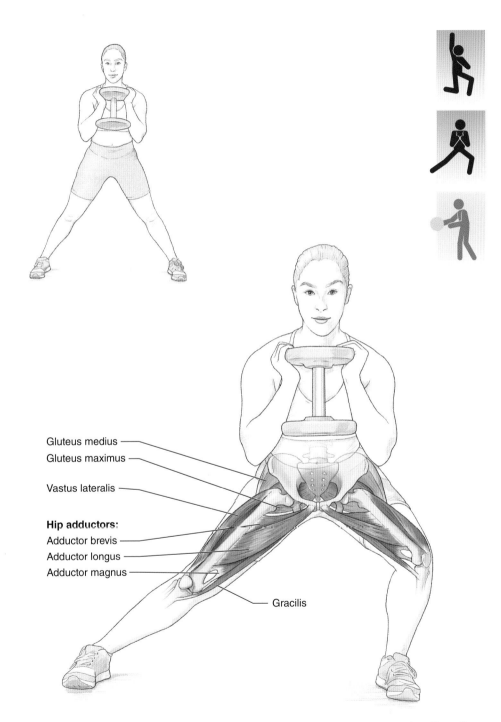

Gluteus medius

Gluteus maximus

Vastus lateralis

Hip adductors:

Adductor brevis

Adductor longus

Adductor magnus

Gracilis

(continued)

GOBLET LOADED LATERAL SQUAT *(continued)*

Execution

1. Stand tall with your legs abducted as far apart as possible, knees straight, feet flat, and toes pointing straight ahead. Hold a dumbbell vertically against your chest with both hands.

2. Descend into a squat downward and laterally to the left while keeping the right knee locked straight. Descend as far as you can while maintaining a flat back and straight right leg.

3. Drive back upward using the glutes and hamstrings. Return to the start position before repeating on the opposite side. Alternate sides until you have completed the programmed repetitions.

Muscles Involved

Primary:

- Hip adductors (adductor longus, adductor magnus, adductor brevis)
- Gracilis
- Vastus lateralis
- Vastus medialis
- Rectus femoris

Secondary:

- Gluteus maximus
- Gluteus medius

FUNCTIONAL FOCUS

The goblet loaded lateral squat is extremely valuable for development of the frontal musculature of the lower body, specifically the adductor muscle group. The adductor muscles are frequently used in sports with frequent cutting and change of direction like soccer, basketball, hockey, and football. Very often weaknesses and underdevelopment of the adductor group can leave these muscles at risk for injury. Training with the lateral squat allows you to place eccentric loaded stress on the adductors in both shortened and lengthened positions, as well as training the gluteus medius and lateral hip stabilizing musculature to aid force generation and stability in the frontal plane.

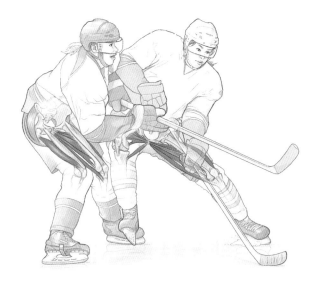

SINGLE-LEG DEADLIFT

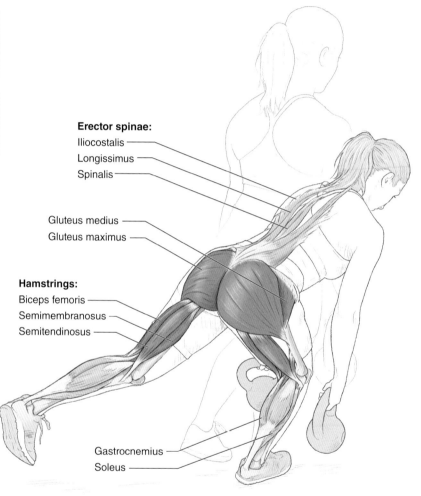

Erector spinae:
Iliocostalis
Longissimus
Spinalis

Gluteus medius
Gluteus maximus

Hamstrings:
Biceps femoris
Semimembranosus
Semitendinosus

Gastrocnemius
Soleus

Execution

1. Begin by standing tall with your feet together and with kettlebells or dumbbells in both hands. Lift your left foot off the ground and begin hinging downward toward the floor. As you hinge, softly bend the right knee so that it is not locked straight. Actively reach the left leg as far back behind you as possible.

2. Once your torso is parallel to the floor, return to the upright position by forcefully contracting the glutes and hamstrings.

3. Perform the programmed number of repetitions and repeat on the opposite side.

Muscles Involved

Primary:

- Hamstrings (semitendinosus, semimembranosus, biceps femoris)
- Gluteus medius
- Gluteus maximus

Secondary:

- Gastrocnemius
- Soleus
- Erector spinae (iliocostalis, longissimus, spinalis)

HIP DOMINANT

(continued)

SINGLE-LEG DEADLIFT   *(continued)*

FUNCTIONAL FOCUS

The single-leg deadlift is a true, functional, posterior chain strengthening exercise when it comes to developing the qualities necessary for sprinting and preventing hamstring strains. The unilateral hinge allows you to eccentrically overload the hamstring muscle group, helping to safeguard it from injury as well as training the hamstrings and glutes to work in concert as hip extensors the way they do during sprinting.

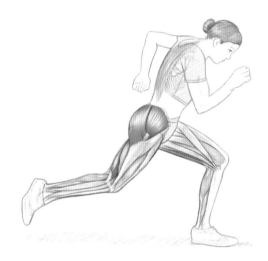

TRAP BAR DEADLIFT

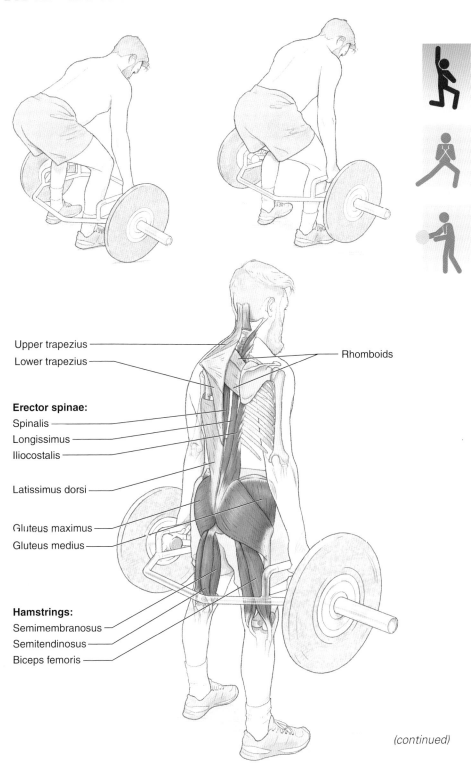

Upper trapezius

Lower trapezius

Rhomboids

Erector spinae:
Spinalis
Longissimus
Iliocostalis

Latissimus dorsi

Gluteus maximus
Gluteus medius

Hamstrings:
Semimembranosus
Semitendinosus
Biceps femoris

(continued)

TRAP BAR DEADLIFT   *(continued)*

Execution

1. Stand inside the trap bar with your feet shoulder-width apart. Hinge downward with a flat spine to the bar and firmly grasp the handles on either side of you. Take a large inhalation and brace your core tightly before beginning the movement.

2. Forcefully extend the hips, using the glutes and hamstrings while maintaining a neutral spinal positioning all the way to the top of the movement.

3. Descend downward, lightly tapping the bar on the ground in between repetitions. Repeat for the programmed repetitions.

Muscles Involved

Primary:

- Hamstrings (semitendinosus, semimembranosus, biceps femoris)
- Gluteus maximus
- Gluteus medius
- Erector spinae (iliocostalis, longissimus, spinalis)

Secondary:

- Vastus lateralis
- Vastus medialis
- Rectus femoris
- Latissimus dorsi
- Rhomboids
- Upper and lower trapezius

FUNCTIONAL FOCUS

The trap bar deadlift should be the main bilateral hip-dominant lift included in a functional sports performance program. High loading potential makes the deadlift a valuable tool for developing full-body strength and hypertrophy in the posterior chain musculature. The patterns trained in the trap bar deadlift translate well to bilateral jumping in sports. The use of the trap bar as opposed to the traditional straight bar makes this exercise easier to teach and reduces the risk of error and injury that can occur with the use of a barbell.

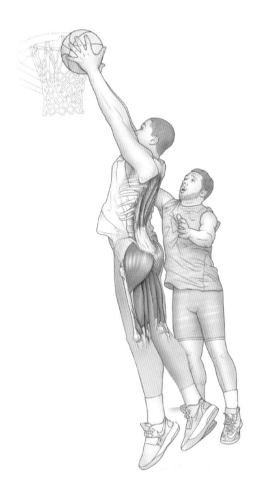

SLIDING LEG CURL

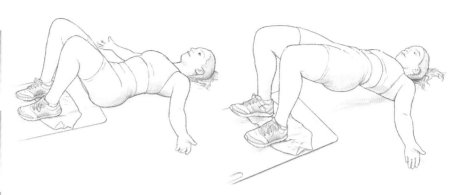

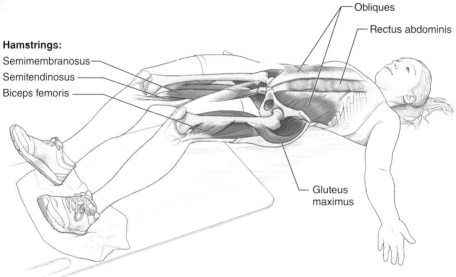

Obliques

Rectus abdominis

Hamstrings:
Semimembranosus
Semitendinosus
Biceps femoris

Gluteus
maximus

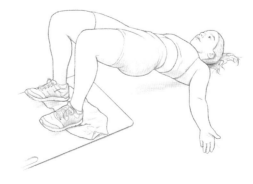

Execution

1. Begin lying in a supine position with your knees bent and hips flexed, with your heels on the ground and ankle and toes dorsiflexed upward. You should perform the exercise with plastic sliders on a turf surface or with a towel on a slide board or hardwood floor so that your feet can slide smoothly.

2. Bridge the hips upward so that the hips are fully extended, creating a straight line from your knees to your shoulders. Slowly begin extending the knees, sliding your feet away from you while maintaining full hip extension.

3. Once the knees are fully extended, reverse direction by actively flexing your knees toward you while driving the hip vertically until you reach the starting position.

4. Maintain braced abdominal muscles and fully extended hips for the entire exercise. Repeat for programmed repetitions.

Muscles Involved

Primary:

- Gluteus maximus
- Hamstrings (semitendinosus, semimembranosus, biceps femoris)
- Obliques

Secondary:

- Erector spinae (iliocostalis, longissimus, spinalis)
- Rectus abdominis

(continued)

SLIDING LEG CURL   *(continued)*

FUNCTIONAL FOCUS

The sliding leg curl trains the hamstrings in concert with the glutes and obliques as they function during sprinting. During optimal sprinting activity, there is a delicate balance between the functions of the hamstrings, glutes, and obliques. There should be coactivation between the hamstrings and obliques to manage the position of the pelvis, as well as coactivation of the glutes and hamstrings to create hip extension. When functioning is optimal, the muscle groups share these tasks to complete the gait cycle. However, when the glutes or obliques aren't functioning properly, the hamstrings become overloaded, often leading to hamstring strains.

This drill trains you to maintain pelvic alignment using the obliques while extending the hips and the glutes and simultaneously taxing the hamstrings with eccentric stress.

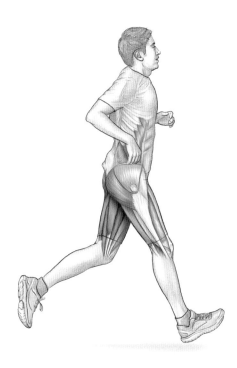

VARIATION

Shoulder Elevated Single-Leg Hip Bridge

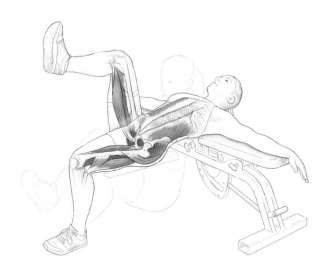

Begin by sitting on the ground with your upper back against a weight bench. Your shoulder blades should be positioned above the top of the bench. Both of your hips should be flexed, with your heels on the floor and your ankles dorsiflexed upward. Flex your right knee as close to your chest as possible, picking your foot up off the floor. Drive the left heel into the floor, actively extending the left hip until the torso is parallel to floor, creating a straight line from your knee to your shoulder. Maintain tension through the anterior core to prevent overextension of the spine. Slowly lower yourself down toward the floor until you touch the ground. Perform the programmed repetitions before repeating on the opposite side.

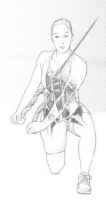

8

CORE AND ROTATIONAL STRENGTH MOVEMENTS

In the mainstream world of fitness and strength training, "core strength" is often associated with the visual appearance of a six-pack abdominal musculature. While having visual abs is a nice aesthetic trait, it has far more to do with one's nutritional routine than it does with the effectiveness of the core muscle function. As seen with bodybuilding, the visual appearance of one's muscles has very little to do with their ability to translate to purposeful function in the athletic arena. The ability to brace and buttress against outside forces, transfer force between the upper and lower extremities, and control the movement of the spinal column is what defines functional core strength.

DEFINING THE CORE

You often hear the word "core" thrown around when people discuss abdominal training, but it is not very often that you see the core defined and broken down into its individual parts. If you are going to train the core musculature effectively, you need to be sure to take the time to accurately define the muscles you should target in the training process.

The core musculature can be broken down into the following muscles:

- Rectus abdominis
- Internal and external obliques
- Transversus abdominis
- Multifidus
- Quadratus lumborum
- Erector spinae (iliocostalis, longissimus, spinalis)
- Diaphragm

All these muscles contribute to overall core strength and stability and should be addressed in a complete functional training program.

"ANTI" CORE TRAINING

Classic core training approaches often feature exercises like crunches and Russian twists that focus on using the core muscles to create motion around the spinal column. While these training methods are widely applied and are effective at creating fatigue in the core muscles, they are misguided in the context of a functional training program.

Functionally speaking, the core muscles work as stabilizers, or anti-movement muscles. Their purpose as it relates to human movement and sport is to buttress the spine, resisting against unwanted motion and assisting in the transfer of force between the upper and lower body.

Core muscles work primarily as isometric and eccentric controllers of motion rather than dynamic and concentric creators of motion.

To ensure effective exercise selection in this chapter, the exercises have been categorized by the movements they prevent rather than the movements they create. Anti-extension and anti-flexion exercises train the muscles that control sagittal plane movement of the spine, rib cage, and pelvis. Anti-rotation exercises train the muscles that control transverse plane motion of the spine, rib cage, and pelvis. Anti-lateral flexion exercises train the muscles that control frontal plane motion of the spine, rib cage, and pelvis.

FRONT PLANK

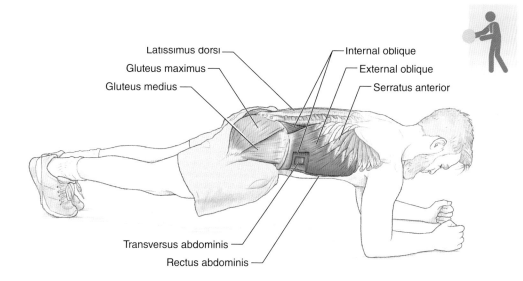

Latissimus dorsi

Gluteus maximus

Gluteus medius

Internal oblique

External oblique

Serratus anterior

Transversus abdominis

Rectus abdominis

(continued)

FRONT PLANK *(continued)*

Execution

1. Begin by lying on the ground in prone position with your elbows under your shoulders and your forearms and fists on the ground. Squeeze your legs together tightly, contract the glutes, posteriorly tilt the pelvis, and draw the rib cage downward.

2. Lift your legs and hips off the ground so that you are supported only by your forearms and feet. Maintain active tension in your abdomen and straight alignment between the sacrum, thoracic spine, and the back of your head.

3. Actively breathe through the nose and out through mouth for the entire exercise to promote abdominal activity. Hold the position for the programmed length of time.

Muscles Involved

Primary:

- Rectus abdominis
- External oblique
- Internal oblique
- Transversus abdominis

Secondary:

- Latissimus dorsi
- Serratus anterior
- Gluteus maximus
- Gluteus medius

FUNCTIONAL FOCUS

Sagittal plane control of the spine, pelvis, and rib cage is foundational to maintaining spinal health as well as efficient force transfer between the upper and lower body. The oblique and rectus abdominis musculature is positioned to depress the rib cage and posteriorly tilt the pelvis, helping to maintain optimal positioning for intra-abdominal pressure. The ability to maintain ideal core and pelvic positioning relieves shearing forces in the intervertebral discs and provides a stable intersection for force transfer between the upper and lower body during athletic movements. The front plank should be the first progression used to train the anti-extension muscles and teach athletes how to maintain optimal sagittal plane positioning.

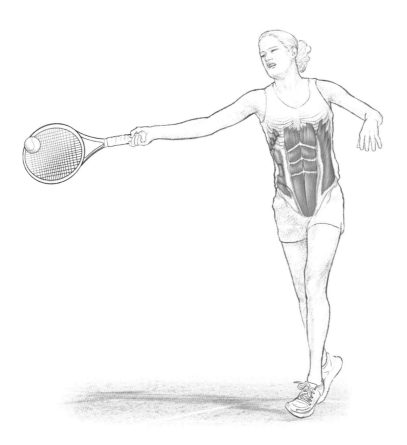

BALL ROLLOUT

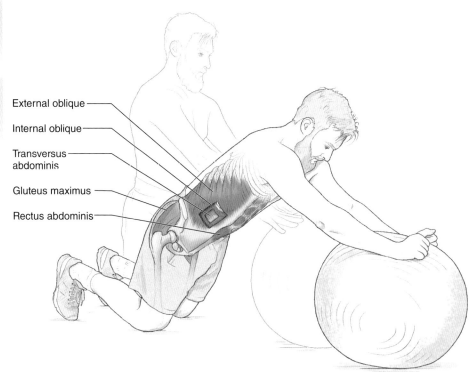

External oblique

Internal oblique

Transversus
abdominis

Gluteus maximus

Rectus abdominis

Execution

1. Begin in a tall kneeling position with your ankle dorsiflexed and toes dug into the ground. Keeping your elbows straight, rest your arms out in front of you on top of a stability ball.
2. Posteriorly tilt your pelvis and draw your ribs downward, maintaining tension in the anterior abdominal wall.
3. Shift your weight forward onto your hands, letting the ball roll forward. Maintain anterior abdominal tension, keeping your head, thoracic spine, and sacrum in a straight line.
4. Roll halfway up the arm before reversing direction and returning to the start position. Repeat for the programmed repetitions.

Muscles Involved

Primary:

- External oblique
- Internal oblique
- Rectus abdominis

Secondary:

- Latissimus dorsi
- Serratus anterior
- Transversus abdominis
- Gluteus maximus

ANTI-EXTENSION

(continued)

BALL ROLLOUT   *(continued)*

FUNCTIONAL FOCUS

The ball rollout is an anti-extension progression to be used following mastery of the front plank exercise. The ball rollout is a more challenging anti-extension variation than the front plank because of the dynamic nature of the exercise and the increased extension force placed on the spine, pelvis, and rib cage. The dynamic nature of the rollout forces you to resist extension and control the static positioning of your trunk in the presence of an increasing extension force as you would have to do during sports.

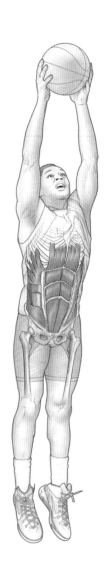

STICK DEAD BUG

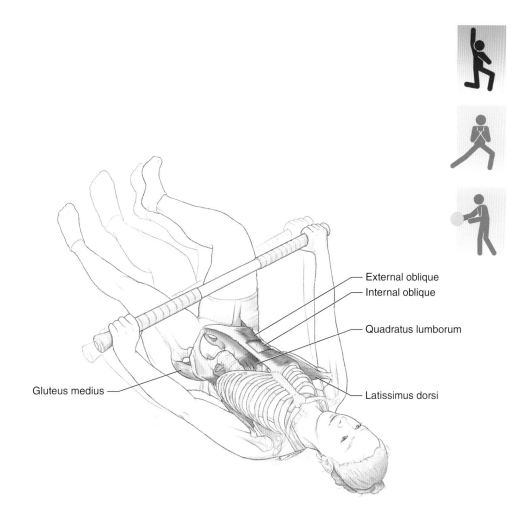

External oblique

Internal oblique

Quadratus lumborum

Gluteus medius

Latissimus dorsi

(continued)

STICK DEAD BUG *(continued)*

Execution

1. Lie on your back with both hips flexed maximally and knees bent. Press a dowel into your thighs with both hands while actively pressing your legs back into the dowel. Maintain your low back pressed into the floor throughout the entire drill.

2. Exhale forcefully, drawing your ribs downward as you extend one leg straight outward. Stop 1 inch (2.5 cm) above the ground before inhaling and returning the leg to the start position.

3. Repeat on the opposite side and alternate sides for the programmed repetitions.

Muscles Involved

Primary:

- Rectus abdominis
- Internal oblique
- External oblique
- Quadratus lumborum

Secondary:

- Transverse abdominis
- Gluteus medius
- Latissimus dorsi

FUNCTIONAL FOCUS

The stick dead bug is a fundamental anti-extension core exercise used to develop sagittal plane control of the rib cage and pelvis. When extending the leg during the drill, you are increasing extension forces on the spine and pelvis, requiring you to create tension in the anterior core musculature to prevent extension. This is representative of the same forces athletes must be able to manage during sprinting to maintain proper running posture.

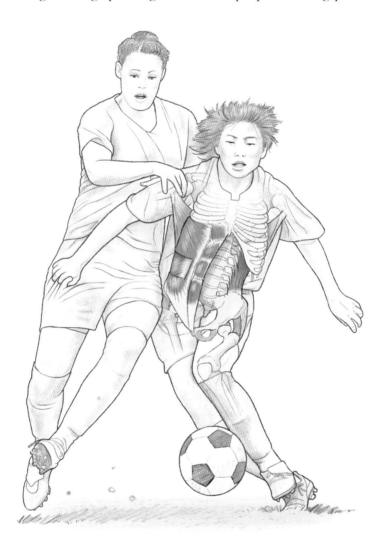

ANTI-ROTATION PRESS-OUT

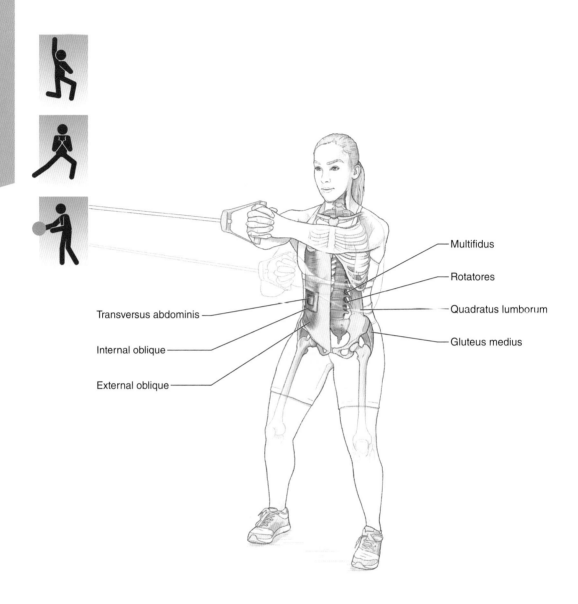

Multifidus

Rotatores

Quadratus lumborum

Gluteus medius

Transversus abdominis

Internal oblique

External oblique

Execution

1. Begin by standing with your feet shoulder-width apart and knees slightly flexed in front of a cable machine. Hold the handle to the cable attachment or band at chest height with both hands, one hand on top of the other.
2. Press the handle straight out in front of you, extending both arms. Resist the pull of the band laterally, bracing your anterior core tight.
3. Return the handle back toward your chest into the starting position. Repeat for the programmed repetitions.

Muscles Involved

Primary:

- External oblique
- Internal oblique
- Multifidus
- Rotatores
- Transversus abdominis

Secondary:

- Gluteus medius
- Quadratus lumborum

(continued)

ANTI-ROTATION PRESS-OUT *(continued)*

FUNCTIONAL FOCUS

The anti-rotation press-out is an isometric rotational exercise. This drill should be used to develop spinal stability and rotational trunk strength in both the reflexive spinal stabilizers (multifidus, transversus abdominis, rotatores) and the prime movers (rectus abdominis, external and internal obliques). During rotational activities the core muscles function less as a producer of motion and more as a transducer of force from the lower body to the upper body. The ability to brace the core and control rotation of the trunk allows you to effectively transfer force from the lower body to the upper body during activities like throwing, punching, striking, and swinging.

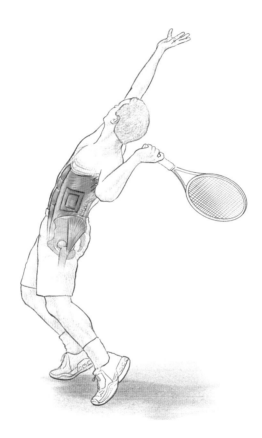

HALF-KNEELING CABLE LIFT

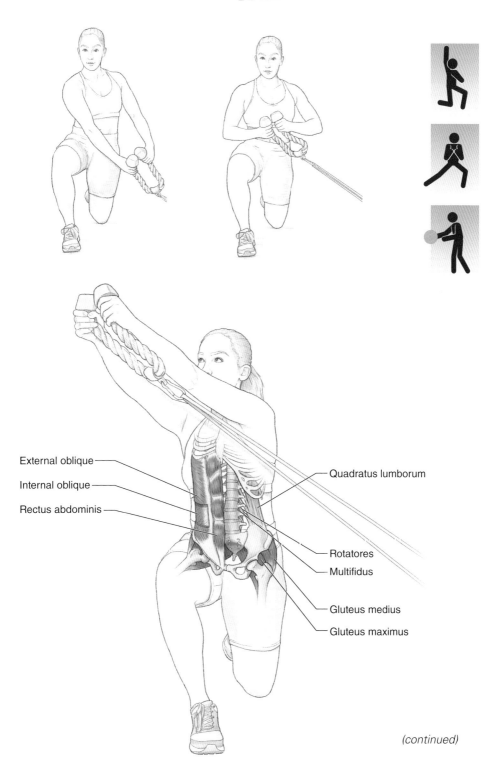

External oblique

Internal oblique

Rectus abdominis

Quadratus lumborum

Rotatores

Multifidus

Gluteus medius

Gluteus maximus

(continued)

HALF-KNEELING CABLE LIFT *(continued)*

Execution

1. Begin in a half-kneeling position with a cable machine or elastic band at your side next to the downside leg. On the kneeling side, dorsiflex the ankle and dig your toes into the ground. Grab the handles to the band or cable with both hands in front of the downside hip with your thumbs facing upward.

2. Pull the handle upward to your chest. Press the handle upward and across your body, extending your arms fully. Lower the handle back down to the starting position, stopping to pause briefly at the chest position again on the way down.

3. Perform the programmed number of repetitions and repeat on the opposite side.

Muscles Involved

Primary:

- External oblique
- Internal oblique
- Rectus abdominis
- Gluteus maximus
- Gluteus medius

Secondary:

- Quadratus lumborum
- Multifidus
- Rotatores

VARIATION

Half-Kneeling Cable Chop

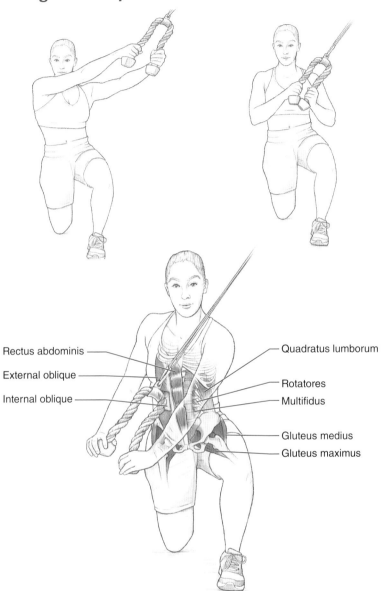

Rectus abdominis

External oblique

Internal oblique

Quadratus lumborum

Rotatores

Multifidus

Gluteus medius

Gluteus maximus

Begin in a half-kneeling position with a cable machine or elastic band at your side next to the upside leg. On the kneeling side, dorsiflex the ankle and dig your toes into the ground. Grab the handles to the band or cable with both hands above the inside hip. Pull the handle down to your chest. Press the handle downward and across your body, extending your arms fully. Bring the handle back up to the starting position, stopping to pause briefly at the chest position again on the way back up. Perform the programmed number of repetitions and repeat on the opposite side.

SUITCASE CARRY

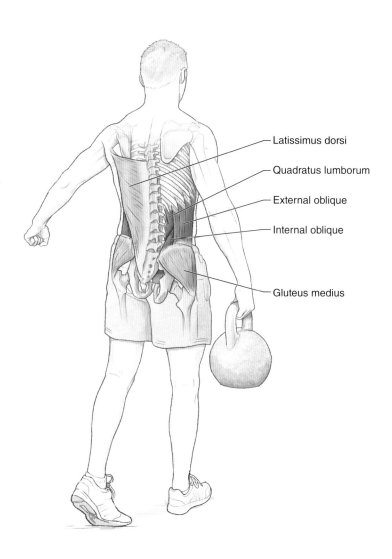

Latissimus dorsi

Quadratus lumborum

External oblique

Internal oblique

Gluteus medius

ANTI-LATERAL FLEXION

Execution

1. Stand tall with a dumbbell or kettlebell in one hand at your side.

2. Walk slowly for the programmed distance, maintaining a tall and even posture without tilting to one side. Actively contract the obliques on the opposite side of the weight to maintain your posture.

3. After walking the programmed distance, switch sides and repeat the exercise.

Muscles Involved

Primary:

- Internal oblique
- External oblique
- Quadratus lumborum

Secondary:

- Gluteus medius
- Latissimus dorsi

(continued)

SUITCASE CARRY *(continued)*

VARIATION

Farmer Carry

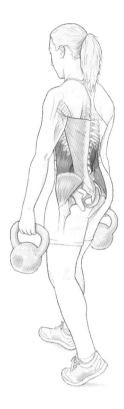

Stand tall with a dumbbell or kettlebell in each hand at your sides. Walk slowly for the programmed distance, maintaining a tall and even posture without tilting, flexing, or extending your spine. Actively contract the lats, obliques, and rectus abdominis to maintain erect posture during the drill. After walking the programmed distance, turn around and walk back to the starting position.

HALF-KNEELING CABLE PUSH-PULL

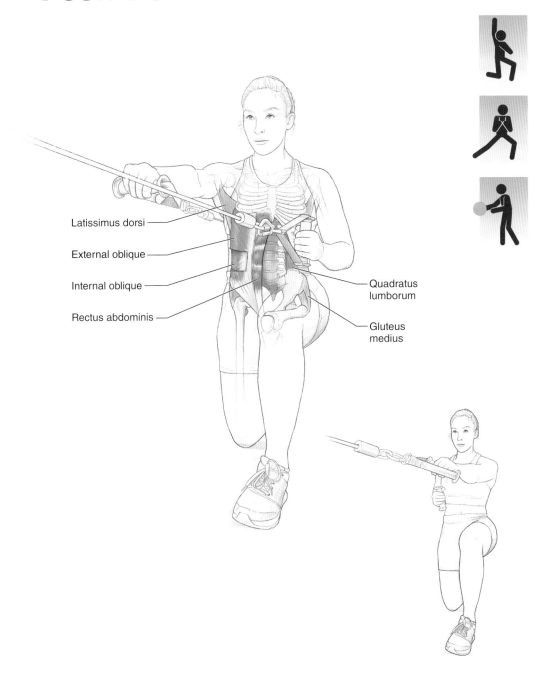

Latissimus dorsi

External oblique

Internal oblique

Rectus abdominis

Quadratus lumborum

Gluteus medius

(continued)

HALF-KNEELING CABLE PUSH-PULL   *(continued)*

Execution

1. Start in a half-kneeling position between two cable machines or resistance bands. On the side where the knee is down, grab the handle that is behind you and position that wrist and forearm at your side next to your rib cage. On the side where the knee is up, grab the handle that is positioned in front of you and outstretch the arm in front of you.

2. Simultaneously, push and pull the handles while resisting rotation at the trunk and keeping your shoulders square ahead.

3. Repeat for the programmed repetitions before switching arms and legs and repeating on the opposite side.

Muscles Involved

Primary:

- Internal oblique
- External oblique
- Rectus abdominis
- Multifidus
- Transverse abdominis

Secondary:

- Gluteus medius
- Quadratus lumborum
- Anterior deltoid
- Triceps brachii
- Latissimus dorsi

FUNCTIONAL FOCUS

The half-kneeling cable push-pull is used to develop sagittal and transverse plane stability in the trunk and frontal plane stability in the hips. This drill rec-reates the torque and stability demands that must be buffered during running. To effectively maintain posture and transfer force down into the ground during gait, you must stabilize rotational forces at the trunk while simultaneously stabilizing the hip and pelvis in the frontal plane. During the push-pull, the focus is to resist the rotational forces of the pushing and pulling motion while keeping the femur and pelvis stacked under the torso in the frontal plane.

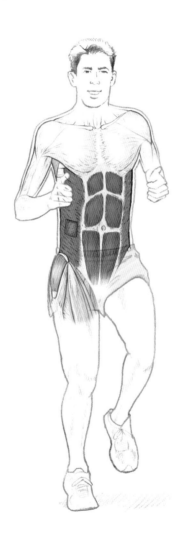

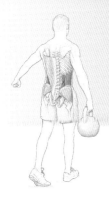

FUNCTIONAL STRENGTH TRAINING PROGRAM EXAMPLES

When designing functional strength training programs, one should strive to build holistic and balanced programs that take into account all the physical stressors of athletic performance. Unlike what occurs with traditional body-building-influenced programming, functional exercise selection should not be based on aesthetic outcomes, but instead on the carryover to the athlete's health and sports performance. The aim is to ensure that the athlete's body is being stressed in all major movement patterns and in all planes of motion to make certain no stone is left unturned in physical development.

A well-balanced program will include exercises from all the categories mentioned in this book. The exercises should be programmed and implemented in the following order to ensure an optimal training outcome:

- Mobility
- Motor control
- Plyometric and medicine ball exercises
- Heavy implement power exercises
- Strength: upper-body push, upper-body pull, hip dominant, knee dominant, anti-extension, anti-rotation, anti-lateral flexion, and anti-flexion

The beginning of the training program should include mobility drills, like active stretching and articular rotations, to improve tissue extensibility and warm up the joints before high-intensity activity. The focus of these drills should be on the ankles, hips, thoracic spine, and glenohumeral joint as these joints frequently exhibit excessive stiffness.

Following mobility work, the next group of exercises in the sequence should be motor control and movement preparation drills. Motor control drills are programmed to activate local stabilizing musculature to improve neurological efficiency and movement quality.

Once you adequately warm up, you can begin participating in high-intensity training activities like plyometric and medicine ball drills. It is important to place high-speed, neurologically demanding movements like hopping, jumping, and throwing early in the program, before strength training, so you will not be performing them while you are fatigued.

After completing plyometric and medicine ball drills, you should progress to the weight room to begin heavy implement power and strength training exercises. The guiding principle is similar to that for programming plyometric and medicine ball drills; you should program heavy implement power drills, like hang cleans and swings, before heavy strength training exercises because of their high neurological demand. To ensure you can perform these exercises at high speed and are not excessively fatigued, cleans, swings, snatches, and sled marches should be performed before exercises such as squats and deadlifts.

It is important to distribute all the strength movement patterns evenly throughout the workout program. Each day should include an exercise from each category: knee dominant, hip dominant, push, pull, and core. Distributing exercise selection in this fashion will ensure you are developing your entire body evenly. The training choices can be broken down easily into the categories shown in table 9.1.

Simply filling in the categories in the chart with some of the exercises covered in this book illustrates how you can categorize exercise selection for simple and balanced programming as in table 9.2.

TABLE 9.1   Exercise Categories

Power	Hip dominant	Knee dominant	Upper push	Upper pull	Core
Heavy implement	Bilateral	Bilateral	Horizontal	Horizontal	Anti-extension
Light implement	Unilateral	Unilateral	Vertical	Vertical	Anti-flexion
					Anti-lateral flexion
					Anti-rotation

TABLE 9.2 Exercise Categories With Exercises

Power	Hip dominant	Knee dominant	Upper push	Upper pull	Core
Barbell hang clean	Trap bar deadlift	Goblet squat	Push-up	Dumbbell row	Front plank
Kettlebell swing	Single-leg deadlift	Split squat	Bench press	Chin-up	Farmer carry
Dumbbell snatch	Sliding leg curl	Single-leg squat	Incline dumbbell bench press	Pull-up	Suitcase carry
Hang snatch			Half-kneeling alternating kettlebell overhead press		Anti-rotation press-out

In the interest of saving time and being efficient, you should look to program all these exercises in pairs or tri-sets, pairing or grouping two or three exercises together and performing them back-to-back in an alternating fashion. It is important to pair or group exercises that are noncompeting, meaning that they are not targeting the same patterns and muscle groups. Creating pairs and tri-sets of noncompeting exercises allows you to be more efficient in that you are training one exercise while simultaneously recovering from another.

Table 9.3 shows an example of a two-day functional training workout routine. Notice how all the exercises in the program are evenly distributed across the two-day program. Both days include equal amounts of hip-dominant, knee-dominant, pushing, and pulling exercises, as well as core and heavy implement power exercises. Beginners should start with the two-day training program to master the basics before progressing to a longer program.

Table 9.4 shows an example of a four-day functional training workout routine. The four-day program is meant for experienced athletes who are physically developed enough to handle increased training frequency. You can see that a four-day workout allows for increased overall training volume as well as greater variety in exercise selection.

TABLE 9.3 Two-Day Functional Training Workout

DAY 1 WORKOUT		
Day 1 movement		
MOBILITY	90/90 Hip stretch	1:00 each side
	Spiderman stretch	1:00 each side
	Straight-leg adductor rocking	10 repetitions each side
	Ankle dorsiflexion	10 repetitions each side
	Shoulder-controlled articular rotation	10 repetitions each side
MOTOR CONTROL	Leg lower with band stabilization	5 repetitions each side
	Floor slide	10 repetitions
	Quadruped hip extension from elbows	5 repetitions each side
	Supine band hip flexion	10 repetitions each side
PLYOMETRIC AND MEDICINE BALL	A1: Hurdle jump	3 sets of 5 repetitions
	A2: Standing medicine ball chest pass	3 sets of 5 repetitions
	A3: 45-Degree bound	3 sets of 5 repetitions each

Day 1 lift		Week 1	Week 2	Week 3	Week 4
HEAVY IMPLEMENT POWER	B1: Barbell hang clean	2 × 5	3 × 5	3 × 5	4 × 3
ANTI-EXTENSION CORE	B2: Front plank	2 × 20 sec	3 × 20 sec	3 × 25 sec	3 × 30 sec
BILATERAL KNEE DOMINANT	C1: Goblet squat	2 × 8	3 × 8	3 × 8	3 × 10
HORIZONTAL PUSH	C2: Push-up	2 × 6	3 × 6	3 × 8	3 × 10
UNILATERAL HIP DOMINANT	D1: Single-leg deadlift	2 × 8 each	3 × 8 each	3 × 8 each	3 × 10 each
HORIZONTAL PULL	D2: Dumbbell row	2 × 8 each	3 × 8 each	3 × 8 each	3 × 10 each
ANTI-ROTATION	D3: Anti-rotation-press-out	2 × 8 each	3 × 8 each	3 × 8 each	3 × 10 each

DAY 2 WORKOUT		
Day 2 movement		
MOBILITY	90/90 Hip stretch	1:00 each side
	Spiderman stretch	1:00 each side
	Straight-leg adductor rocking	10 repetitions each side
	Ankle dorsiflexion	10 repetitions each side
	Shoulder-controlled articular rotation	10 repetitions each side
MOTOR CONTROL	Leg lower with band stabilization	5 repetitions each side
	Floor slide	10 repetitions
	Quadruped hip extension from elbows	5 repetitions each side
	Supine band hip flexion	10 repetitions each side
PLYOMETRIC AND MEDICINE BALL	A1: Single-leg hurdle hop	3 sets of 5 repetitions each
	A2: Standing medicine ball side toss	3 sets of 5 repetitions each
	A3: Overhead medicine ball throw	3 sets of 5 repetitions each

Day 2 lift		Week 1	Week 2	Week 3	Week 4
HEAVY IMPLEMENT POWER	B1: Barbell hang clean	2 × 5	3 × 5	3 × 5	4 × 3
ANTI-EXTENSION CORE	B2: Front plank	2 × 20 sec	3 × 20 sec	3 × 25 sec	3 × 30 sec
BILATERAL HIP DOMINANT	C1: Trap bar deadlift	2 × 8	3 × 8	3 × 8	4 × 6
VERTICAL PULL	C2: Chin-up	2 × 5	3 × 5	3 × 5	3 × 6
UNILATERAL KNEE DOMINANT	D1: Two-dumbbell loaded split squat	2 × 8 each	3 × 8 each	3 × 8 each	3 × 10 each
VERTICAL PUSH	D2: Half-kneeling alternating kettlebell overhead press	2 × 6 each	3 × 6 each	3 × 6 each	3 × 8 each
ANTI-LATERAL FLEXION	D3: Suitcase carry	2 × 40 yd each	3 × 40 yd each	3 × 40 yd each	3 × 40 yd each

TABLE 9.4 Four-Day Functional Training Workout

DAY 1 WORKOUT		
Day 1 movement		
MOBILITY	90/90 Hip stretch	1:00 each side
	Spiderman stretch	1:00 each side
	Straight-leg adductor rocking	10 repetitions each side
	Ankle dorsiflexion	10 repetitions each side
	Shoulder-controlled articular rotation	10 repetitions each side
MOTOR CONTROL	Leg lower with band stabilization	5 repetitions each side
	Floor slide	10 repetitions
	Quadruped hip extension from elbows	5 repetitions each side
	Supine band hip flexion	10 repetitions each side
PLYOMETRIC AND MEDICINE BALL	A1: Hurdle jump	3 sets of 5 repetitions each
	A2: Standing medicine ball chest pass	3 sets of 5 repetitions each

Day 1 lift		Week 1	Week 2	Week 3	Week 4
HEAVY IMPLEMENT POWER	B1: Barbell hang clean	2 × 5	3 × 5	3 × 5	4 × 3
ANTI-EXTENSION CORE	B2: Front plank	2 × 20 sec	3 × 20 sec	3 × 25 sec	3 × 30 sec
BILATERAL KNEE DOMINANT	C1: Goblet squat	2 × 8	3 × 8	3 × 8	3 × 10
HORIZONTAL PUSH	C2: Push-up	2 × 6	3 × 6	3 × 8	3 × 10
BILATERAL HIP DOMINANT	D1: Sliding leg curl	2 × 6	3 × 6	3 × 8	3 × 10
HORIZONTAL PULL	D2: Dumbbell row	2 × 8 each	3 × 8 each	3 × 8 each	3 × 10 each
ANTI-ROTATION	D3: Anti-rotation press-out	2 × 8 each	3 × 8 each	3 × 8 each	3 × 10 each

DAY 2 WORKOUT		
Day 2 movement		
MOBILITY	90/90 Hip stretch	1:00 each side
	Spiderman stretch	1:00 each side
	Straight-leg adductor rocking	10 repetitions each side
	Ankle dorsiflexion	10 repetitions each side
	Shoulder-controlled articular rotation	10 repetitions each side
MOTOR CONTROL	Leg lower with band stabilization	5 repetitions each side
	Floor slide	10 repetitions
	Quadruped hip extension from elbows	5 repetitions each side
	Supine band hip flexion	10 repetitions each side
PLYOMETRIC AND MEDICINE BALL	A1: Single-leg hurdle hop	3 sets of 5 repetitions each
	A2: Standing medicine ball side toss	3 sets of 5 repetitions each

Day 2 lift		Week 1	Week 2	Week 3	Week 4
HEAVY IMPLEMENT POWER	B1: Kettlebell swing	2 × 10	3 × 10	3 × 10	4 × 10
ANTI-EXTENSION CORE	B2: Stick dead bug	2 × 20 sec	3 × 20 sec	3 × 25 sec	3 × 30 sec
HORIZONTAL PUSH	C1: Barbell bench press	2 × 8	3 × 8	3 × 6	4 × 6
UNILATERAL HIP DOMINANT	C2: Single-leg deadlift	2 × 8 each	3 × 8 each	3 × 10 each	3 × 10 each
VERTICAL PUSH	D1: Half-kneeling alternating kettlebell overhead press	2 × 6 each	3 × 6 each	3 × 8 each	3 × 8 each
UNILATERAL KNEE DOMINANT	D2: Goblet loaded lateral squat	2 × 6 each	3 × 6 each	3 × 8 each	3 × 8 each
ANTI-ROTATION AND ANTI-EXTEN-SION	D3: Half-kneeling cable chop	2 × 8 each	3 × 8 each	3 × 10 each	3 × 12 each

(continued)

(Table 9.4 Four-Day Functional Training Workout continued)

DAY 3 WORKOUT		
Day 3 movement		
MOBILITY	90/90 Hip stretch	1:00 each side
	Spiderman stretch	1:00 each side
	Straight-leg adductor rocking	10 repetitions each side
	Ankle dorsiflexion	10 repetitions each side
	Shoulder-controlled articular rotation	10 repetitions each side
MOTOR CONTROL	Leg lower with band stabilization	5 repetitions each side
	Floor slide	10 repetitions
	Quadruped hip extension from elbows	5 repetitions each side
	Supine band hip flexion	10 repetitions each side
PLYOMETRIC AND MEDICINE BALL	A1: 45-Degree bound	3 sets of 5 repetitions each
	A2: Sprint start chest pass	3 sets of 5 repetitions each

Day 3 lift		Week 1	Week 2	Week 3	Week 4
HEAVY IMPLEMENT POWER	B1: Barbell hang clean	2 × 5	3 × 5	3 × 5	4 × 3
ANTI-EXTENSION CORE	B2: Front plank	2 × 20 sec	3 × 20 sec	3 × 25 sec	3 × 30 sec
BILATERAL HIP DOMINANT	C1: Trap bar deadlift	2 × 8	3 × 8	3 × 8	4 × 6
VERTICAL PULL	C2: Chin-up	2 × 5	3 × 5	3 × 5	3 × 6
UNILATERAL KNEE DOMINANT	D1: Single-leg squat	2 × 5 each	3 × 5 each	3 × 8 each	3 × 8 each
HORIZONTAL PUSH	D2: Push-up	2 × 6	3 × 6	3 × 8	3 × 10
ANTI-FLEXION	D3: Farmer carry	2 × 40 yd	3 × 40 yd	3 × 40 yd	3 × 40 yd

DAY 4 WORKOUT

Day 4 movement

MOBILITY	90/90 Hip stretch	1:00 each side
	Spiderman stretch	1:00 each side
	Straight-leg adductor rocking	10 repetitions each side
	Ankle dorsiflexion	10 repetitions each side
	Shoulder-controlled articular rotation	10 repetitions each side
MOTOR CONTROL	Leg lower with band stabilization	5 repetitions each side
	Floor slide	10 repetitions
	Quadruped hip extension from elbows	5 repetitions each side
	Supine band hip flexion	10 repetitions each side
PLYOMETRIC AND MEDICINE BALL	A1: Explosive step-ups	3 sets of 5 repetitions each
	A2: Rotational one-arm chest pass	3 sets of 5 repetitions each

Day 4 lift		Week 1	Week 2	Week 3	Week 4
HEAVY IMPLEMENT POWER	B1: Kettlebell swing	2 × 10	3 × 10	3 × 10	4 × 10
ANTI-EXTENSION CORE	B2: Stick dead bug	2 × 20 sec	3 × 20 sec	3 × 25 sec	3 × 30 sec
HORIZONTAL PUSH	C1: Incline dumbbell bench press	2 × 8	3 × 8	3 × 8	4 × 8
UNILATERAL KNEE DOMINANT	C2: Rear foot elevated split squat	2 × 6 each	3 × 6 each	3 × 8 each	4 × 8 each
ANTI-ROTATION	D1: Half-kneeling cable push-pull	2 × 8 each	3 × 8 each	3 × 10 each	3 × 12 each
UNILATERAL HIP DOMINANT	D2: Shoulder elevated single-leg hip bridge	2 × 6 each	3 × 6 each	3 × 8 each	3 × 10 each
ANTI-ROTATION AND ANTI-EXTENSION	D3: Half-kneeling cable lift	2 × 8 each	3 × 8 each	3 × 10 each	3 × 12 each

EXERCISE FINDER

MOBILITY EXERCISES

90/90 Hip Stretch (External Rotation and Flexion Focus)	14	
90/90 Hip Stretch (Internal Rotation and Extension Focus)	16	
Spiderman Stretch	17	
Straight-Leg Adductor Rocking	20	
Half-Kneeling Hip Flexor Stretch	23	
Wall Quad Stretch	26	
Ankle Dorsiflexion	29	
Shoulder-Controlled Articular Rotation (Flexion Focus)	32	
Shoulder-Controlled Articular Rotation (Extension Focus)	34	

(continued)

MOTOR CONTROL AND MOVEMENT PREPARATION EXERCISES

Supine Diaphragmatic Breathing	38	
Floor Slide	41	
Wall Slide	44	
Leg Lower With Band Stabilization	45	
Unassisted Leg Lower	48	
Quadruped Hip Extension From Elbows	49	
Supine Band Hip Flexion	52	

PLYOMETRIC AND MEDICINE BALL EXERCISES

Hurdle Jump	59	
45-Degree Bound	62	
Lateral Bound	64	

HEAVY IMPLEMENT POWER EXERCISES

(continued)

HEAVY IMPLEMENT POWER EXERCISES (*continued*)

Dumbbell Snatch	93	
Sled March	96	

UPPER-BODY STRENGTH EXERCISES

Push-Up	102	
Half-Kneeling Alternating Kettle-bell Overhead Press	105	
Barbell Bench Press	108	
Incline Dumbbell Bench Press	111	
Chin-Up	114	
Pull-Up	116	
Dumbbell Row	117	

LOWER-BODY STRENGTH EXERCISES

Goblet Squat	124	
Rear Foot Elevated Split Squat	127	
Two-Dumbbell Loaded Split Squat	129	
Single-Leg Squat	130	
Goblet Loaded Lateral Squat	133	
Single-Leg Deadlift	136	
Trap Bar Deadlift	139	
Sliding Leg Curl	142	
Shoulder Elevated Single-Leg Hip Bridge	145	

(*continued*)

CORE AND ROTATIONAL STRENGTH MOVEMENTS

ABOUT THE AUTHORS

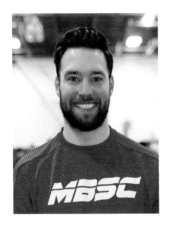

Kevin Carr is a strength and conditioning coach and manager at Mike Boyle Strength and Conditioning (MBSC) as well a massage therapist and cofounder of Movement as Medicine, a massage and movement therapy clinic in Woburn, Massachusetts. He is the cofounder of the Certified Functional Strength Coach certification. He has a bachelor's degree in kinesiology from the University of Massachusetts at Amherst and a license in massage therapy from Cortiva Institute in Watertown, Massachusetts.

Carr amassed a wealth of experience in the field of sport performance and personal training while working at MBSC and has traveled all over the world to educate thousands of coaches and therapists about the MBSC coaching system. He has coached everyone from U.S. Olympians looking for a competitive edge to the average person looking to shed some pounds, move better, and improve their health.

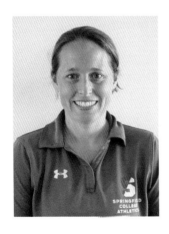

Mary Kate Feit, PhD, is an assistant professor of strength and conditioning in the School of Physical Education, Performance, and Sport Leadership at Springfield College in Massachusetts. At Springfield College, she also serves as the associate director of strength and conditioning, overseeing the graduate assistant strength and conditioning coaches, who serve over 600 student-athletes at the college. Prior to her work at Springfield College, she had an extensive career in sport performance, which included time spent as an assistant strength and conditioning coach at the University of Iowa and the University of Louisville as well as the adult program coordinator at Reach Your Potential Training in Tinton Falls, New Jersey.

Feit completed her graduate degree in applied exercise science with a concentration in strength and conditioning from Springfield College and her bachelor's degree in biology from the College of the Holy Cross, where she was a Division I soccer player. Her love for strength and conditioning originated when she began sport performance training under fellow Springfield alum Mike Boyle at Mike Boyle Strength and Conditioning (MBSC), where she spent seven summers coaching athletes while finishing her high school and collegiate education. She is certified through the National Strength and Conditioning Association, Collegiate Strength and Conditioning Coaches Association, Precision Nutrition, and Functional Movement Systems, and she holds the Certified Functional Strength Coach designation.

ANATOMY SERIES

Each book in the *Anatomy Series* provides detailed, full-color anatomical illustrations of the muscles in action and step-by-step instructions that detail perfect technique and form for each pose, exercise, movement, stretch, and stroke.

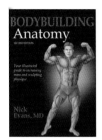 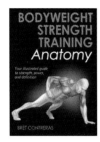 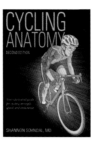 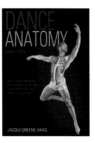 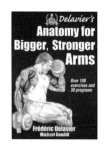

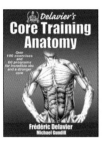 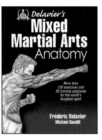 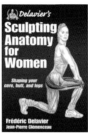 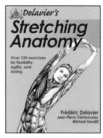 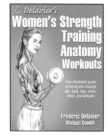

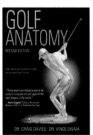 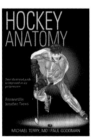 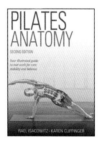 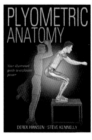 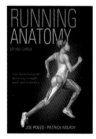

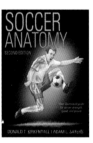 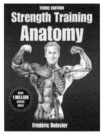 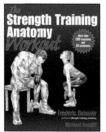 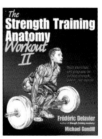 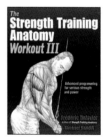

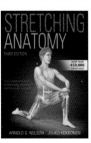 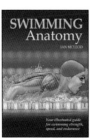 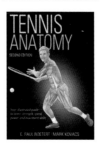 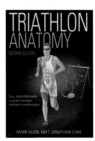 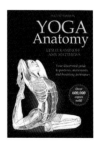

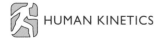

U.S. 1-800-747-4457 • US.HumanKinetics.com/collections/anatomy
Canada 1-800-465-7301 • Canada.HumanKinetics.com/collections/anatomy
International 1-217-351-5076

You read the book—now complete the companion CE exam to earn continuing education credit!

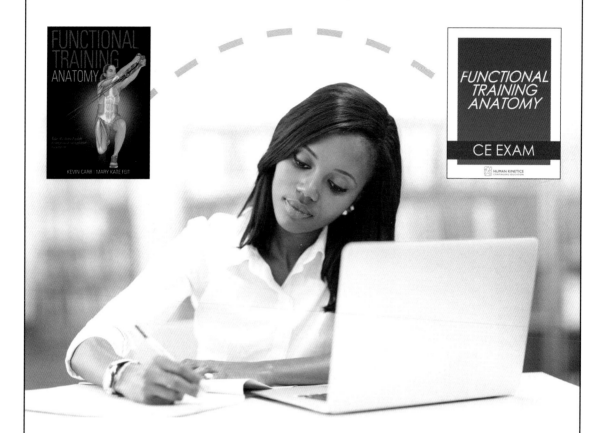

Find and purchase the companion CE exam here:
US.HumanKinetics.com/collections/CE-Exam
Canada.HumanKinetics.com/collections/CE-Exam

50% off the companion CE exam with this code

FTA2022

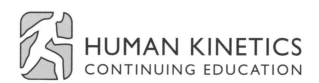